What if You Were Thin?

The Kaizen Program for
Permanent Weight Loss!

By Rachel D. Young

改善

Author's Note

The exercises and advice contained within this book may be too strenuous or dangerous for some people, and the reader(s) should consult a physician before engaging in them.

Always consult your physician or other health-care provider before beginning any exercise, nutritional or weight-loss program, especially if you suffer from a bad back, heart disease, or other medical problem or condition. If you're going to engage in weight-training exercise, I recommend that you consult with a licensed fitness trainer or expert.

The author and publisher of this book are not responsible in any manner whatsoever for any injury which may occur through reading and following the instructions herein.

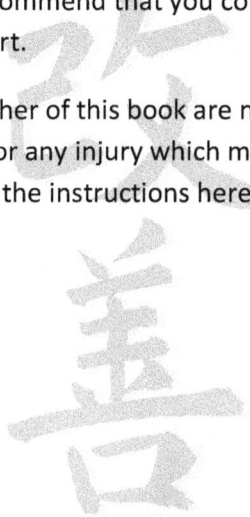

改善

Praise for "What If You Were Thin"!

"As Editor in Chief of a site with over 300,000 daily unique visitors, I see *all* the fad diets, the instant weight loss pills, and the unrealistic expectations people put on themselves to lose weight. Rachel Young's unique book, What if You Were Thin and her one-of-a-kind Kaizen method is a realistic way to lose weight and keep it off! If you're tired of gaining and losing the same weight over and over again, you should buy What if You Were Thin!"

Kris Gethin

:: Editor-In-Chief

www.bodybuilding.com

"After six months...you'll feel like you need a satellite dish to track how far you've traveled. You'll feel light years ahead of the game. Most importantly, you'll realize that you took control over an issue that seemed impossible to resolve. Without pushing yourself to do more faster, you can and will arrive at the place you've wanted to be all along."

Matt Furey

Tampa, FL

Fitness Professional

www.MattFurey.com

"You have inspired and motivated me. If you think the only way to lose weight is to go away to a "Biggest Loser Ranch"...all anyone needs to do is to follow you, Rachel. I look to you and what you've been able to teach and think it's simply amazing. You're really making a difference."

Pete Thomas

NBC's Biggest Loser

At-Home Winner, Season 2

www.WhatIfYouWereThin.com

"The method for weight loss that Rachel teaches is one I've advocated for years. Its one of the safest and most reliable in existence today. Rachel takes the confusion out of eating to make weight loss easy for anyone. I highly recommend it!"

Dr. Keith-Thomas Ayoob
Associate Clinical Professor at the Albert Einstein College of Medicine
Director of the Nutrition Clinic at the Rose F. Kennedy Children's Evaluation and Rehabilitation Center

"I am SO glad I bought 'What If You Were Thin.' After reading the book and watching Rachel's videos, I can tell you that she is witty, insightful, intelligent, encouraging and a motivator. She will help you ask yourself the right questions and get to the bottom of your weight problem once and for all. If you are ready to change your life, get this book. It's not a 'get skinny FAST' program. You will not empty all of your cabinets the first day, spend $500 at the store on chemical-laden, fat free products, pre-packaged meals and shakes that may make you SKINNY, but they'll kill your kidneys, liver and other parts of your body. You will not run to the store and spend tons of money on workout equipment that eventually ends up under your bed where you constantly stub your toes on them and remember that you are not only over weight, but a quitter too. What you WILL do is slowly, one step at a time, change your life. She will meet you where you are and guide you through creating new habits in fitness and in eating healthy foods that not only help you lose weight, but will nourish your mind and body as well. I'm down 10 pounds so far and THIS time, it's staying off!"

Erin Strowbridge
Birmingham, AL

www.WhatIfYouWereThin.com

What if You Were Thin? The Kaizen Program for

Permanent Weight Loss!

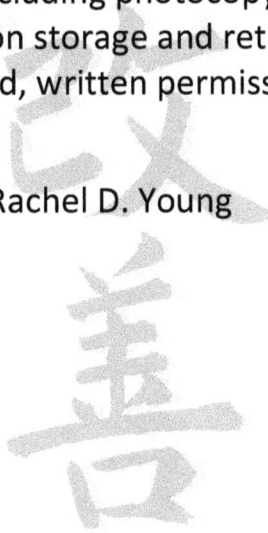

改善

This book is Dedicated:

To my selfless husband John: "Thank you" will never be enough.

To my children, Charlotte, Chandler, and KJ: One day you'll look back on all the crazy days of writing, editing, and will understand that everything I do is because of you.

To the overweight adult reading this book: It's never too late. It's never too much. It's never too far. You can do this. I believe in you!

改善

Foreword for
What if You Were Thin?

Throughout my career as a wrestler, martial artist and fitness professional, I cannot begin to count how many times I've dealt with people who wanted to lose all their excess weight "yesterday." You know who I'm talking about, right?

Quick weight loss is the normal way of thinking in our society. Instead of following the ages old *natural* admonition to "make haste slowly" – most people try to "make haste quickly." And before long no haste is being made at all, except what appears to be excessive weight gain.

Mark my words, as someone who is also guilty of years of quick weight loss in the sporting world, I can unequivocally say that "normal" may be the "norm" ... but it is not natural, nor does it last. When you do the normal thing, you may enjoy temporary quick-fix results, but never a truly positive lasting change.

The natural way to healthy weight loss is to coax your body to make progress. When you are coaxed bit by bit, there's no snap-back or rebounding effect because you introduced changes to your life in an evolutionary rather than a revolutionary manner. Your mind and body can accept incremental changes but they have a difficult time with radical changes. Too much too fast and every cell in your body revolts, recoils and regains whatever weight you've lost.

The above is part of the reason why I'm so excited to endorse John and Rachel Young's book *What if You Were Thin?* Instead of preaching the typical hurry-up approach to weight loss or the dull and boring western method of only keeping tabs, they've given the unique twist to weight loss that western minds can truly benefit from and use. And that twist is the Kaizen Method of improving your eating, your exercising and your health. It's undoubtedly worked miracles for John and Rachel, and I believe it will for you, too, if you simply do what they recommend.

After six months to a year of following the supposedly slow method of incremental improvement, you'll feel like you need a satellite dish to track how far you've traveled. You'll feel light years ahead of the game. Most importantly, you'll realize that you took control over an issue that seemed impossible to resolve. Without pushing yourself to do more faster, you can and will arrive at the place you've wanted to be all along.

Enjoy your journey!

Matt Furey
www.mattfurey.com

Table of Contents

改善

What Condition Are You In?

Take the following test to see if The Kaizen Program is right for you!

1. Do you feel yourself 'dragging' in the afternoon, losing energy?
2. Do you feel older than you are?
3. Do you try to use bulky clothes to hide your figure?
4. Are you stressed?
5. Do you feel depressed?
6. Do you get sick often?
7. Do you have lower back and neck pain?
8. Do your muscles feel sore, even though you don't exercise?
9. Do you feel beaten up when you wake up in the morning?
10. Do you feel like you have no control over your life?
11. Do you have a hard time waking up?

12. Do you have a hard time going to sleep?

13. Who gets tired first, you or the kids?

14. Does your boss complain about your lack of productivity after lunch?

15. Would you rather have a root canal than join a gym?

If you answered yes to any of these questions, then The Kaizen Program was made for you!

You Are in the Right Place!

You have made the best decision of your life. You've become a member of the Kaizen family! By joining the team, you've made the choice to better your life and potentially those around you as well.

Here are just a few of the many benefits you'll start to receive from studying and implementing the **The Kaizen Program**:

1. The flab hanging over your belt will disappear (and your hips, thighs, chin(s)...wave them all goodbye)!

2. You'll sleep better at night and find it easier to get up the next morning.

3. You'll discover a boost in self-confidence and esteem that could lead to promotions you never expected to receive.

4. You'll buy fewer antacids because you'll have better digestion and an increase in circulation.

5. Others in your life (and the office) will become easier to get along with (test us on this one. You'll find we're right!)

6. You'll start off keeping us to yourself but once the weight begins to come off, you'll want the whole world to know!

7. You'll have an increase in energy like never before (Those afternoon naps will be a thing of the past forever)!

改善

Rules, Comments, and Instructions

Rule #1: Be ok with being sore – you're using muscles that may have been ignored for a while. You're going to ache in a few new places. It's alright. You're doing something good for your body.

Rule #2: Don't let clowns derail you – "Keep away from those who try to belittle your ambitions. Small people always do that, but the really great make you believe that you too can become great." - Mark Twain

Rule #3: No Whining! – This is something positive you're doing for your life and it should stay that way! Whining gives a negative association to the positive changes you're making in your body!

Rule #4: No excuses – You don't have to get up early or rearrange your schedule, buy equipment, or pay outrageous membership dues. You've got no one to blame but yourself if you don't do the work.

Rule #5: Strive for progress, not perfection – Life isn't perfect and neither are you. Work on getting it right 'most of the time' and more often than not, you'll find good things happen to your body!

Rule #6: It's OK to be human – Similar to #5, but not the same. While you want to make progress on this plan, there will be office parties or birthday party cake will be involved. It is perfectly fine to eat a slice and not feel guilty at all. You're human. Enjoy life or else what's the point?

Rule #7: Take it personally – This is about you and your body. Not your neighbor, not your boss. Take this personally and make it work for you. If you don't take care of yourself, everyone else will have to when you're too fat and crippled to do anything about it.

Rule #8: See yourself at your best – Visualize the progress you want to make. Get pictures from magazines or on the internet of what you want to achieve (be realistic). Put them up everywhere to remind yourself of what you're working towards.

Rule #9: Reward yourself – While healthy, longer life is its own reward, you still gotta give yourself something along the way. A new outfit, some new running shoes, maybe even a long weekend away. Just make sure the reward isn't going to set you back on your goals.

Rule #10: Track your results – At the end of this book you'll find a worksheet you can use to track your weight loss and health goals. Print it out and use it as often as you need to in order to achieve the goals you've set for yourself.

You can do this! I believe in you!

Part I – Introduction to Kaizen

改善

Chapter 1: "What is Kaizen?"

*H*ow many diets have you tried that were solely devoted to getting you thin within a specific amount of time? It was all microwave-fast. *Get thin quick.*

But they were probably based on you doing-without-something-you-love, eating like a bird, and generally asking the impossible of you. And what happened when you stopped following the diet? Chances are, you not only gained back what you'd lost, but you packed on a few extra pounds as well!

As certified physical trainers and nutrition junkies, my husband and I both wondered about what truly made people thin...forever? The one's that stuck with the program, the ones that "got it"...what made them stay that way? Why did one particular program "work" – was it the program or the mind of the person following it? What kept them from putting the weight back on?

For years, I'd struggled with my own weight and had repeatedly been unsuccessful with any diet, pill, or plan I'd tried.

This was more than a curiosity about the opposite of weight *LOSS*. What did those who dropped the weight GAIN in return?

This curiosity, plus an interest in shedding 150 pounds between my husband and I, lead to the book you're now reading.

But I'm getting ahead of myself. My introduction to *kaizen* – the catalyst for my own dramatic weight loss, actually took place many years ago...

Rachel Meets Kaizen

Growing up in Japan as a child of missionary parents; *kaizen* was a way of life for me. I barely remember any different.

You see, the Japanese use the term *"kaizen"* to describe small steps that can be taken to achieve large goals. I used this concept to learn the language (speaking and writing), to try and discover new local foods, to live and love the country I was being raised in.

So, what exactly *is* "kaizen"?

According to Wikipedia, the term kaizen (改善, Japanese for "good change") is a Japanese word adopted into English referring to a philosophy or practices focusing on continuous improvement in manufacturing activities, business activities in general, and even life in general, depending on interpretation and usage. When used in the business sense and applied to the workplace, kaizen typically refers to activities that continually improve all functions of a business, from manufacturing to management and from the CEO to the assembly line workers.

By improving standardized activities and processes, kaizen aims to eliminate waste (see lean manufacturing). Kaizen was first implemented in several Japanese businesses during the country's recovery after World War II and has since spread to businesses throughout the world. (*Source: Wikipedia*)

The original kanji (Chinese characters) for this word are: 改 善

In Japanese this is pronounced "*kaizen*".

• 改 ("kai") means "change" or "the action to correct".

• 善 ("zen") means "good".

Hence, kaizen means "good change".

I spent over 7 of the most formative years of my teenage life observing Japanese culture, customs, and integrating my own behavior to become as close to Japanese as I could get. The kaizen way of thinking became almost second nature to me...but it wasn't always like that.

I had to learn slowly. I had to make changes as they came. It was just like learning to ride a bike all over again – the Japanese way. Learning the train system, how to order food, asking for directions. These all took time to make them a way of life as natural as waking up each morning.

But by the time I was 15, I couldn't imagine life any differently! I ate Japanese food. I rode the train an hour to school each day. I spoke Japanese (even with my friends who spoke fluent English)! My favorite pastime was to go to the local karaoke bar with my friends and sing until we were too hoarse to go any further.

On special holidays, like Bon Odori, I even dressed in the traditional Japanese yukata (similar to a kimono, but not as formal).

Yes, life in Japan was good. But as they say, "all good things must come to an end" and the day after I graduated from high school, I was on a plane, headed for the next big change in my life...college.

Life as a Fat Chick

Once in college, the fast-paced lifestyle that we Americans enjoy quickly became my new way of life. There were some adjustments to be made to fit in stateside, but I adapted and soon the kaizen way of thinking was a thing of the past.

I rediscovered the joy of drive-thru windows, of convenience stores, of junk food. I re-learned the guilty pleasures of going out to get a chocolate bar in the middle of the night, just because I wanted one.

I never felt bad about it, though. I'd often run into my friends at the same convenience store in the wee hours of the morning doing the same thing I was – buying junk!

Years went by and I put on more weight with each passing year. I met a man in college and got married – and things went downhill from there. I woke up one morning to find myself overweight, a full time college student with a new baby, and two full time jobs.

I never slept. I ate whatever was in reach whenever I had a spare second to do so. "Exercise" was the energy I used to get from the car to the next job and make it through the day. I smoked like a chimney as it was often the only way I could stay awake driving to my next job or class.

I was so unhappy.

After the birth of my 3 children, a failed marriage, and facing a 90 pound weight-gain from years of poor eating habits (*and who has time for exercise*???), I became easily overwhelmed with the thought of getting the weight off and keeping it that way!

So I began my search for the "magic pill" that would cure my fatness. Diets, weight loss drinks, pills, you name it – I tried it!

Laxatives
Diet pills
Counting points
Counting calories
Liquid diets
Fruit diets
Colonic flushes

The list went on and on. I'd try anything once!

I just wanted a quick fix – something to help me wake up one morning, happy with my body and the skin I was living in.

I was always looking for something to make it all better. Even trips to the supplement store! I'd joke with my husband John that, "if the store manager says, '*Hey, we just got these magic pills in. I thought you'd wanna try them. Lose 50 pounds overnight!*' then we're getting them!"

But of course, he never said that. And I never found my 'magic pill'. Just a bunch of caffeine pills and money-wasters.

Problem was, nothing worked. Any weight I lost while taking a pill came right back when I stopped.

Any weight loss from eating some 'low calorie', 'low fat', or 'no sugar added' food was short-lived.

I'd usually get hungry afterwards and binge on something that was the complete opposite of what I should be eating.

Then I'd feel guilty, go back to what I should'a been eating, and the cycle would start again. Sometimes I'd get so depressed I'd skip the 'what I shoulda been eating' part and went straight to the binge.

It was a depressing cycle and something had to be done fast!

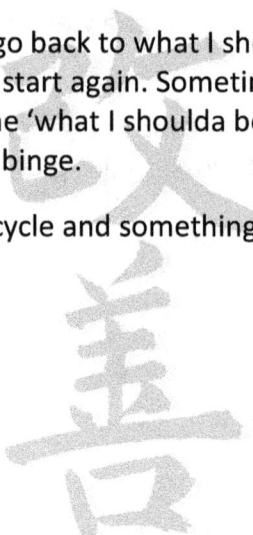

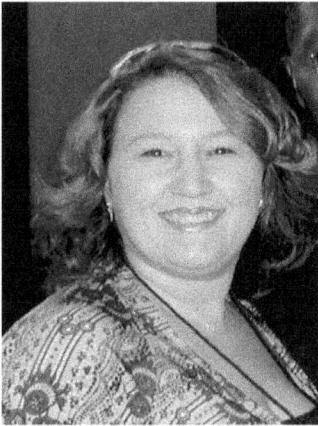

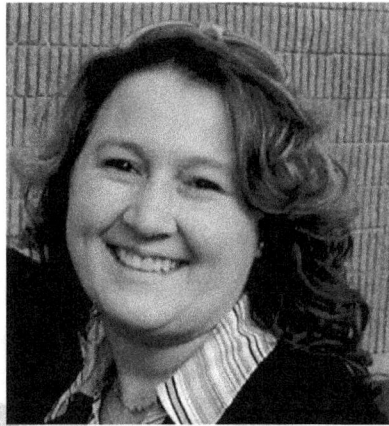

**Smiling on the outside – crying on the inside.
At 210 pounds, I was a heavy girl!**

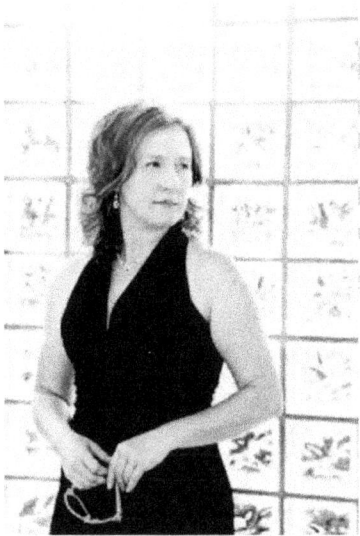

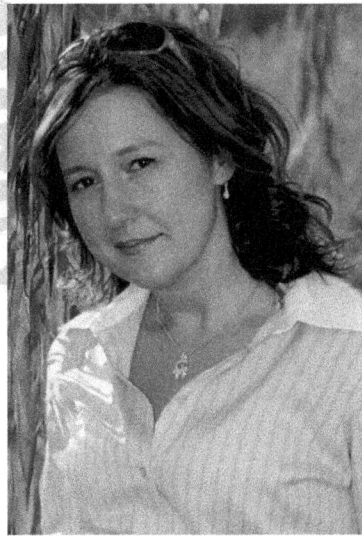

**What a difference 80 pounds makes!
At 130, I'm a much happier lady!**

改善

Chapter 2: How Does Kaizen Apply to Weight Loss?

After years of binging and dieting, trying every weight loss pill on the planet, or exercising until I was too sore to move for a week, I'd resigned myself to the fact that I was never gonna be thin. I would never wear a size 6. I would never be the skinny girl I was in high school.

Fortunately, I was very, very wrong. I'm currently a size 4 and will tell you how I got that way in just a few pages. But first, I had to realize I was fat!

My First Aha Moment
My 'Aha moment' came first. I attended a seminar where I would get to meet (for the first time, face-to-face) the mentor I credited with providing me with business-growth

and educational information necessary to take my copywriting business to great heights.

I was overjoyed at the thought of getting to shake hands with the man whom I deemed responsible for my success. I wanted to shower him with compliments, gush over how much I appreciated his help, to show my appreciation for his willingness to share his knowledge and experience with me.

The day came. I saw my opportunity to talk with one of the two men I wanted to meet. The batteries in my camera died as we prepared to have our picture taken together – what a missed opportunity! Fortunately someone else stepped in and snapped the photo.

Weeks later, I got an email with the photo attached. And when I opened the picture, I was mortified.

Why had this person sent me a picture of someone else? That wasn't me! That was a picture of someone who didn't care what she looked like. Who ate like a cow, smoked like a factory, and had 'checked out of life'.

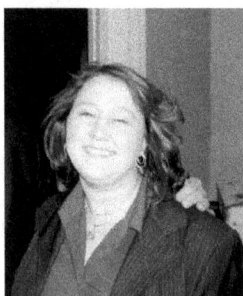

Oh…my…gosh – **THAT PICTURE WAS OF ME!**

But that couldn't be! Was this really the image I wanted to show to the world? That I'd checked out? That I didn't care? That wasn't true!

I decided right then and there that SOMETHING had to be done.

But no magic pills this time. No more roller coaster. This had to be permanent.

Taking the First Step

That day, I decided to have a salad with my lunch. It was still loaded with cheese, bacon bits, creamy ranch dressing, and croutons. But it was a salad. And that was the point.

I enjoyed it so much, I did it again the next day. And the next. And the next. And after a week, I enjoyed having salads with my lunch and decided to keep having them.

Mind you, I still ate cheeseburgers and fries. I just added a salad to my meal. And not every meal. Just the one at lunch.

Two weeks later, I decided to add a salad to dinner as well.

No big change. Just a little salad at lunch and dinner. Not a big deal. I could take it or leave it. It just so happened that I enjoyed it and decided to keep the salads around.

Remember, I was piling the salad up with bacon, creamy ranch dressing, and enough other toppings to easily eat my daily caloric intake in that one dish.

But it was a salad and that was a good step in the right direction for me.

And I think this is how permanent weight loss should start for everyone. With one small step.

- Throw away the first bite of your favorite chocolate bar.
- Have a salad with your lunch. Don't try to make it super healthy. Just as long as there's lettuce involved. ☺
- Park at the back of the parking lot when you go to the grocery store.

Little things that can add up to big results!

That's how the Kaizen Program is gonna get the weight off you for good. One small, itty bitty step at a time.

You realize you didn't put the weight on overnight and that's not how you're gonna lose it.

You put it on one bite at a time and we'll take the weight off of you together – one bite at a time FOREVER. You will never be fat again when you're following this program!

Recipe for Permanent Weight Loss

If someone tasked you with creating the World's Best Chocolate Soufflé, you wouldn't throw a bunch of ingredients you'd never heard of into a bowl and proclaim that you're done, right?

The same holds true for your weight loss.

We aren't gonna throw a bunch of exercises and some unrealistic meal plan at you and declare that you're gonna be thin tomorrow. This stuff takes time and unless you take the time to make these changes *permanent*, when you're finished with this book, you'll go right back to the exact same eating habits that made you heavy in the first place.

In fact, statistics show you'll gain even more weight after a failed diet attempt! That means this Kaizen plan is gonna stick and become permanent.

The only dish I ask you to bring to this party is Patience. Be willing to take the weight off slowly and you'll see some surprising results, namely:

- When you lose weight slowly, you're less likely to have loose, saggy skin afterwards!

- You're more likely to keep the weight you lose off for longer!
- You'll be able to recognize and eliminate cravings and binges by taking the time to learn about what triggers these reactions in your body!

This is the last "diet" book you'll ever buy – because we're gonna create a new lifestyle for you, not just an eating plan!

From this point on, I don't want you to even think about trying a 24-hour all-grapefruit plan, a magic pill to eliminate subcutaneous water from your body, or spending 3 hours in the gym so you can eat a piece of cake without guilt.

Starting today, we're going to make small, subtle changes so that this really sticks for you. You've seen that I've lost over 80 pounds on my blog (www.whatifyouwerethin.com) and I KNOW that by making these little steps the program will work for you as well.

This isn't about having nasty meals delivered to your house that are the portion size of a Happy Meal!

We're going to do away with One Diet Fits All and create a customized plan that will not only work for you, but anyone else you want to help along the way!

To Sum It Up

1. You didn't get this way overnight and won't lose the weight overnight. Be patient!
2. This is about changing your lifestyle, one step at a time. Don't do anything radical or it won't "stick"!
3. Don't worry. I'm gonna be here the whole way to help you out. Remember, I went through this 80+ pounds ago and know exactly what you're going through!

改善

Chapter 3: Why the Kaizen Method WILL Help You!

*Y*ou're above the whole "magic pill" idea.

You know that diet and exercise is the key, but who wants to throw their schedule into chaos, spend hours in the gym, and sit around eating lettuce all day long?

From here on out, you're gonna begin, step-by-step, to make subtle, small changes in your daily life and begin to see BIG results very, very quickly!

Not starting Monday. Not tomorrow. Today! Right now!

Using these small, Kaizen steps, you'll slowly but permanently incorporate healthy eating choices and fitness goals so that they become as common in your lifestyle as getting dressed in the morning.

You don't think about the fact that you put clothes on. You just do it. Sure, you pick out what you're gonna wear, just like you'll pick out your food and choose your workout each day – but the act of eating, doing, and living a Kaizen life will become 2nd nature to you!

This is gonna mean the difference between dreading your High School Reunion and anxiously anticipating it.

It means you won't be embarrassed to wear a swimsuit, regardless of the season!

It means that you can finally eat in public without fear that people are commenting about your food choices behind your back.

We'll begin your journey to a healthy body with Three Basic Steps to Your Kaizen Body:

- Kaizen Eating (with Beginner and Advanced Stages)
- Kaizen Fitness (with 3 different workouts for varied lifestyles)
- Kaizen Life (for when life happens!)

In this next chapter, we'll take a broad overview to each one, then get into the nitty gritty! Don't skip ahead! I put these chapters in order for a reason! Take it one step at a time!

Chapter 4: Three Basic Steps to Your Kaizen Body

*I*n order to make small steps towards positive change, you gotta have a plan, a path to take, goals to work towards.

The Kaizen Program is broken up into three basic steps and will get you to your goals faster, easier, and healthier than you ever thought possible!

Step 1: Kaizen Eating. We'll cover what to eat and when, how to eat at any food joint and not feel guilty, and how to overcome cravings.

You'll see recipes you can make yourself, specific tips and tools to keep from returning back to your old way of eating, and even specific meals during the week that allow you to eat WHATEVER YOU WANT!

Step 2: Kaizen Fitness. You'll discover a variety of workout programs that fit your current lifestyle, no alterations necessary, without joining a gym, buying expensive equipment, or breaking your back to get a workout in! In fact, you can do some of these exercises directly in front of a co-worker or spouse and they'll never even know you're working out!

Who says you gotta spend a lot of money, get primped up to go to the gym, and feel self-conscious that people are watching you work out? You can do these moves in front of them and never feel like you're under a microscope!

Step 3: Kaizen Life. It happens. Cravings attack. You set goals and miss them. You have days that you just want a cheeseburger, fries, and a shake. Together we'll walk through the steps to handling each of these obstacles and coming out a winner!

At the end of some chapters, you'll see a section entitled "To Sum It Up". Here, I'll summarize the main points from that chapter (and have included them in a chapter at the end for you to print and use as guidance whenever you need a little boost)!

Now – enough talking! Let's get started!

Part II - Kaizen Eating

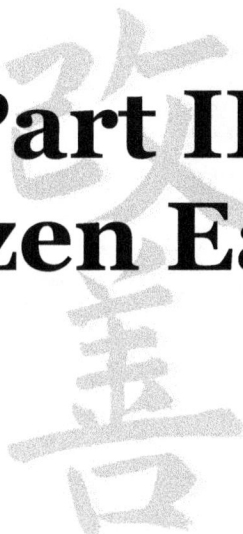

改善

Chapter 5: Your Brain and Its Chemicals

W hy start out the eating chapter by talking about stress?

First of all, if you're human, chances are you eat when you're stressed. There's a reason for this, which we'll get to in a minute.

Most importantly, stress is easily 70% of the reason you're struggling with your weight right now!

I'll explain:

Back in the 'olden days' when man lived in caves and hunted saber-toothed tigers for food, nature equipped him with a beautiful system.

You see, sometimes man hunted for food, and sometimes the food got the better of the man and he had to get away – fast!

Nature devised a system by which man, when he needed to, could call upon stored energy reserves to either "fight or flight" – either stand his ground or get the heck outta there!

You know them as HORMONES.

Going Hormonal

Norepinephrine, epinephrine, and cortisol are all released by your adrenal glands whenever you're faced with "certain peril" (i.e. getting away from that saber-toothed tiger that didn't die when you shot him with an arrow).

Norepinephrine and epinephrine cause several changes to help you survive the danger, including a pause in insulin release so you have lots of blood sugar available for energy, an increase in heart rate and blood pressure, and a suspension of your appetite.

The Cortisol Effect

After the danger has passed, cortisol tells the body to stop producing norepinephrine and epinephrine and stimulates your appetite again.

But what happens when there's no "tiger" to get away from?

What happens when the stress at work is on you 24/7, when you have looming deadlines, traffic to fight, kids to feed, or other stressors that never stop?

The cortisol just sits in your blood, building up with nowhere to go.

Cortisol turns into fat, increasing your cravings for high-fat, high-carb foods.

And when you give into those cravings and the brain steps in again.

This time, the brain unleashes chemicals, specifically serotonin, dopamine, and opiate peptides. These chemicals are positioned at optimal levels for positive mood and euphoric feelings.

In plain English, when you eat, they make you feel good.

Combining a high-stress lifestyle with the euphoria of eating and you've got a recipe for obesity that is sweeping the United States at an alarming rate!

A potentially-dangerous addiction to food begins to develop that, if left unchecked, can lead to obesity and worse!

Artificial Sweeteners

Now you're trying to justify yourself by whining, "I only drink *Diet* Coke! I only eat *No Sugar Added* stuff! Why do I still have a weight problem?"

Here's a little more 'science' for ya regarding aspartame, saccharine, sucralose, cyclamate, and acesulfame K.

As it stands, saccharine presently carries a government mandated warning label that it is known to cause cancer in laboratory animals.

Aspartame is broken down in the body to wood alcohol, subsequently broken to formaldehyde, a fixative and a known carcinogen (cancer causing agent). Formaldehyde is then broken down into formic acid, which is the same strong caustic used by fire ants to administer their sting.

Most recently, a Purdue University study released in the journal Behavioral Neuroscience showed that rats given artificial sweeteners gained more weight than rats given the real thing. Why?

One simple word: Insulin.

The Skinny on Insulin

You often hear about 'insulin' as it applies to diabetics. Perhaps you've felt the effects of it when you're blood-sugar levels have gotten too high or low (hyper- or hypoglycemia).

When you consume anything (food, drink, etc) your body begins the digestion process. There are several "traffic cops" along the way, telling the food and resulting nutrients where to go and how to get there.

One such "traffic cop" is insulin.

Insulin directs the sugar in the food you've eaten to various organs, including your liver.

When you ingest an artificial sweetener, the brain (aka head honcho) sends a message downstream, "Hey! We're eating sugar! Get the insulin ready to send this stuff where it needs to go!"

The pancreas responds by creating massive amounts of insulin. Insulin then waits for an onrush of sugary traffic.

When the artificial sweetener hits your stomach, insulin levels increase due to the perceived demand for glucose in your blood stream (our bodies turn it into energy).

Over time, this leads to insulin resistance within the body and can potentially lead to...***pre-diabetes!***

The Zero Calorie Lie

A calorie is a unit of heat equal to the amount of heat required to raise the temperature of one kilogram of water by one degree at one atmosphere pressure (Source: Wikipedia).

It is physically IMPOSSIBLE for anything you put in your body to have zero calories. The diet drinks, the diet foods, the gum, the snacks – they all have to go somewhere and they all have to be either used, stored, or eliminated by the body in some fashion.

The truth is that, thanks to artificial sweeteners like those listed earlier, your body is being tricked into believing that you're receiving something sweet and reacting accordingly (remember those rewarding brain chemicals?)

The Bottom Line

The meal plans in the following chapter will include few (if any) artificial sweeteners (Stevia is ok in my book).

And if you need a degree in Advanced Physics to read the label – you won't find it in any of our recipes!

All you need is a few minutes of preparation and the right ingredients to keep your office meals (and home too) on the road to good health (and a great body!)

To Sum It Up

1. If you can't reduce the stress in your life (or find a better way to handle it), you'll have a hard time losing the last few pounds due to cortisol.
2. Artificial sweeteners create an illusion within the body that insulin is needed and can eventually cause "insulin resistance" (and lead to diabetes).

3. There's no such thing as "zero calories" – regardless of what the label says!

Chapter 6: Meal Planning

*I*t's Sunday. Tomorrow you're heading back to the office and the thought of going through one more drive-thru window makes you cringe.

But who has time to make a week's worth of great meals that aren't gonna break the budget or leave you rushing to eat because it took too long to prepare? YOU DO!

Starting today, we're gonna change the way you look at meals forever! The recipes and meal plans on the following pages are gonna be just the thing you're looking for to get you to a healthier, happier body – fast!

Since your working hours aren't the ONLY time you're going to eat, I've included some simple dishes you can have ready for breakfast or dinner that the rest of the family can enjoy without throwing you off course!

What to Look For

There are several keys we'll look for in a good recipe (and then, of course, we'll give you the recipes!)

First, and most importantly, the foods you choose to eat must be "clean".

That means, nothing processed, nothing hard-to-pronounce, nothing that uses every word in the alphabet to spell.

Second, in order to get your food into the package and onto the store shelves, if anything more than a knife has touched it, you don't want it.

No 'special packaging machinery' please!

In other words, you want as little human interaction with your food as possible so that we know you're getting the freshest, most nutritious food possible!

If you can't order it lean from the butcher, pick it, or grow it – you don't eat it.

Third, remember that you're human! Sometimes life happens: kids' birthdays, office parties, holidays...things come up where it's OK to have a piece of cake or have a soda with your meal (we'll talk about your special 'cheat' meals in a minute).

You didn't get this way from eating a cupcake and you won't gain anything back from eating one every once in a while. Moderation is now the name of the game!

Finally, choose meals that can perform 'double duty'. For example, the recipe we use for Ginger Chicken can easily be converted to a Ginger Chicken Wrap for lunch the following day.

Cooking less often but still healthy and nutritious meals will make losing the weight at work easier than you think! In fact, most of your meals can be prepared in less than 10 minutes if you plan ahead!

For dinner, try a short marinade of lemon and teriyaki sauce. Select some thinly sliced steak from the local grocery store (mine cost about $7.00 for a package and that feeds both my husband and I for two nights!) You can also consider some thinly sliced pork chops (boneless will cook faster).

A package of pre-sliced veggies like red and green peppers, onions, and mushrooms round out this meal, keep it clean and lean, and can all be done on a George Foreman-type grill in less than 10 minutes.

So which would you rather have: a steak from a restaurant that you wait an hour to get a seat, wait an additional 30 minutes to get your food, and then pay **$35 for two people** to eat (plus the added sodium, fat, and other culinary factors beyond your control)...or spend 10 minutes and approximately **$3 per person** and KNOW what went into your food because you put it there???

You can use the recipes laid out in the following chapter, but you certainly don't have to! The grocery store is a wonderland of choices and opportunities – enjoy it!

Keep in mind that you'll probably want to pick up a food scale from Bed, Bath, and Beyond or Tuesday Morning. It can be a real eye-opener when you see just how much food makes one portion for you vs. what you've actually been putting on your plate. That's half the battle right there!

For your meat, stick with approximately 3-4oz per main meal (if you're eating out, that's about the size of your fist). For your side items (which we'll talk about more in the next few chapters), stick to 2oz, or about the size of your palm.

Now you've got your measuring cup wherever you go, so no more excuses!

To Sum It Up:
1. Look for "clean" food – if you can't pronounce it's ingredients, can't grow it, pick it, or get it cut lean from your butcher, don't eat it!
2. You're human. Birthday cake is ok as long as it's only a slice and only a rare occasion.
3. Cut your grocery bill by buying fresh and eating in rather than paying someone else to cook for you!

So, with the rules laid out, let's talk recipes!

Chapter 7: Kaizen Recipes

Breakfast:

Banana Nut Pancakes
On *Sunday night*, mix together:

1 cup oatmeal
¾ cup crushed pineapple
4 egg whites (approx. ¾ cup)
1 scoop whey protein powder
¼ cup finely chopped walnuts (or pecans)
dash o' cinnamon
splash o' vanilla
2Tbsp organic sugar (or Stevia)

Refrigerate overnight (or if you forgot to make it the night before, let it sit for 10 min before cooking.)

For breakfast, drop ¼ cup of the mixture into a hot skillet over medium heat (be sure to use your favorite non-stick organic cooking spray!)

Cook the pancake on each side until golden brown.

Make 2 pancakes for yourself and garnish with a chopped banana.

One batch should make 3 meals worth and is safe to store in the fridge for that amount of time.

Just make sure to make your next batch on Wednesday night!

Power Shake
30g whey protein powder
8 oz water (or fat-free milk if you absolutely must)
½ cup oatmeal (soak overnight for a lighter consistency)

(Add a tablespoon of flaxseed for added fiber and "good fat")

Better-Than-Poptarts
2 sliced Ezekiel bread (or your choice of whole grain bread)
1 Tbsp natural peanut butter

Add an egg on the side, cooked the way you like it (no cheese) for added protein.

Egg and Sausage Sandwich
4 egg whites
1 oz veggie sausage
1 toasted whole-wheat English muffin

Cook per the directions then eat with a side of strawberries (1 cup).

Apple Butter Oatmeal
¾ cup oatmeal, instant
½ scoop whey protein isolate, vanilla
1 cup water
1 cup apple, sliced
1 tbsp. natural peanut butter

Place oatmeal and water in a microwaveable bowl. Stir, slowly adding in the protein powder until completely mixed. Cook on high for approximately 1-2 minutes. Add peanut butter and apple slices. Stir and serve.

Raisin French Toast Bites
2 slices Ezekiel raisin bread
4 egg whites
3 tbsp. low-fat milk
Dash of cinnamon

Preheat a large skillet over medium heat. In a large shallow bowl, mix together the egg whites, milk, and cinnamon. Lightly dip the bread pieces in the mixture and place on skillet. Brown each slice for about 3-4 minutes (flip about halfway through cooking time), and then serve. You may also try topping it with fresh fruits, yogurt, or cottage cheese. Even light maple syrup! Serves one.

Lunch:

Classic Turkey Sandwich
1 toasted whole-wheat English muffin
3 fresh deli turkey slices or vegetarian turkey slices
2 medium slices tomato,

1 tsp hummus
15 baby carrots (as a side)

Stack together in sandwich form and yummy in your tummy!

Fruit Infused Chicken Salad
3 cups spinach
3 oz boneless, skinless grilled chicken
1 wedge Laughing Cow Light cheese
½ cup sliced strawberries
8 walnut halves
2 tbsp vinaigrette

Combine and grab a fork!

Asian Veggie Patties Done Right!
1 Morningstar Asian Veggie Patty
½ cup brown long grain rice
4-5 stalks bokchoy (Chinese cabbage)
1 tbsp Teriyaki sauce

Lightly brown the patty in your favorite nonstick pan. At the same time, prepare the rice for your lunch the next day! Add the teriyaki sauce right before you're ready to take the patty out of the pan. Add the bokchoy to the empty saucepan with a Tbsp of water to slightly wilt. Combine all the ingredients in a bowl and enjoy!

Classic Tuna Sandwich
4 ox canned tuna
1 tbsp hummus
lettuce leaf
1 slice tomato
1 slice onion
2 slices multigrain Ezekiel bread

Combine and eat with 15 grapes as a side dish for lunch. Wanna have it for dinner? Leave off the bread and eat on a bed of romaine lettuce instead!

Better Than Subway
2 slices whole wheat bread
3 slices deli-sliced turkey breast
fresh bell pepper slices
fresh red onion slices
large handful of spinach
2 slices of tomato

Combine everything together and enjoy! The bread is just something to hold all of those yummy veggies together!

Can be made ahead of time to enjoy at the office or a perfect summertime lunch!

Dinner:

Pork Fajita Casserole
(Prep time is 30 minutes. Total time is 60 minutes)

1 large red onion, halved, sliced lengthwise
½ red bell pepper, sliced into 1 ½-inch strips
½ green bell pepper, sliced into 1 ½-inch strips
2 tsp canola oil
1 lb lean pork cutlet, sliced into 2-inch strips
3 large cloves garlic, sliced
1 tbsp cumin
2 ½ tsp chile powder
½ tsp ground black pepper
3 medium low-fat whole-wheat tortillas, divided
1 15-oz can black beans, drained, rinsed, and divided
2 tomatoes, chopped and divided

½ cup baby spinach, divided
¼ cup low-fat cheddar cheese, shredded
½ avocado, diced

Preheat oven to 350°F.

In a large skillet, sauté onion and bell peppers in oil for 5 minutes over medium-high heat. Add pork, garlic, and seasonings. Cook for 8 minutes.

Prepare casserole: In an 8x8 inch clear glass dish, begin to layer ingredients. Place 1 tortilla on bottom and add ¼ of pork-vegetable mixture, 5 oz black beans, ¼ cup tomatoes and ¼ cup spinach. Continue with second tortilla, following with the same order of ingredients and amounts. Sprinkle cheese over top layer. Bake for 20 to 25 minutes, until top is bubbly. Let cool for 5 to 10 minutes. When serving, top each casserole piece with 2 tsp avocado. Best enjoyed within 4 to 5 days. Store in fridge in an airtight container.

Ginger Chicken
12 oz boneless, skinless chicken breast
½ tbsp olive oil
1 tsp minced garlic
1 tbsp chopped fresh ginger
1 medium onion, cut into wedges
1 large red bell pepper, cut into strips
2 cup broccoli florets
½ cup reduced-sodium chicken broth, divided
1 tsp arrowroot powder
2 tbsp low-sodium soy sauce
2 cups brown rice, cooked

Slice chicken into strips. Heat oil in a large skillet over medium-high heat; add chicken and sauté about 5 minutes. Remove and set aside.

Add garlic, ginger, onion, pepper, broccoli, and ¼ cup chicken broth. Saute for 5 minutes. Meanwhile, stir arrowroot powder into the remaining chicken broth and add soy sauce.

Return chicken to pan, add soy sauce mixture and bring to a boil. Stir, until sauce thickens slightly. Cook 1 minute longer.

Serve half the chicken without the brown rice for dinner, reserving the rice plus the remaining chicken and veggies until the following day.

Note: This recipe does DOUBLE DUTY!

The day after you have Ginger Chicken for dinner, grab the leftover chicken and veggies on your way out the door to work.

During lunch, reheat the chicken, and enjoy!

Turkey Cutlets Dijonnaise
1.3lb turkey breast cutlets
1 large egg
¾ cup wheat germ
¼ cup grated low-fat Parmesan cheese
½ cup Greek yogurt
1 tbsp Dijon mustard

Preheat oven to 400°F. Place cutlets between two long pieces of plastic wrap and pound gently with fist to flatten.

Meanwhile, scramble egg with a little bit of water in a shallow bowl and mix wheat germ and Parmesan on a large plate.

Soak each cutlet in egg mixture, then dredge in wheat germ mixture before placing on a cooling rack set over a cookie sheet.

Bake for 15 minutes or until no longer pink, flipping halfway through. Combine yogurt and mustard and spoon over cooked cutlets.

Desserts:

"Ice Cream" Sandwiches
1 recipe Vanilla Frozen Yogurt (see below)
1 recipe Chocolate-Spiked Oatmeal Cookies (see below)

Instructions:
To assemble sandwiches, spoon 3 tbsp frozen yogurt between 2 cookies. If yogurt is too hard to scoop, allow it to warm slightly for a few minutes on counter until desired consistency. Repeat for remaining cookies. Eat immediately or transfer to freezer-safe container and store in freezer until ready to eat. For best results, eat within 2 to 3 hours of filling cookies.

Vanilla Frozen Yogurt
1 ½ cups strained low-fat plain yogurt
¼ cup agave nectar
2 tsp pure vanilla extract

In a mixing bowl, combine strained yogurt, agave and vanilla. Stir until well blended, then spoon mixture into a shallow 9x9-inch non-reactive freezer-safe container.

Transfer container to freezer and chill until mixture is starting to freeze slightly around the edges, about 45 minutes. Scrape ice crystals from edges with a spatula and mix thoroughly back into yogurt mixture. Continue to blend until creamy again, about 2 minutes. Return container to freezer and repeat this process 2 more times, for a total of 3 times. Each time the mixture will get thicker and a little harder to blend. After the third mixing, return container to freezer until ready to eat, about 2 to 3 hours. For best results, store tightly sealed in freezer and use within 2 to 3 days.

Chocolate-Spiked Oatmeal Cookies
Olive oil cooking spray
1 ¼ cup quick-cook old-fashioned oats
½ cup whole-wheat pastry flour
2 tsp flaxseed meal
1 tsp cinnamon
½ tsp baking powder
¼ tsp sea salt
½ cup agave nectar
1 large egg white
2 tsp unsalted almond butter
1 tsp pure vanilla extract
¼ cup dark bittersweet chocolate chips

Preheat oven to 350°F and lightly spray 2 baking sheets with cooking spray.

In a large mixing bowl, combine oats, flour, flaxseed meal, cinnamon, baking powder and salt.

In a small mixing bowl, whisk together agave, egg white, almond butter and vanilla.

Add egg mixture to dry ingredients all at once and combine. Stir in chocolate chips.

Divide batter equally into 16 mounds (about 1 rounded tbsp in size) and arrange evenly spaced on prepared baking sheets. Using the back of a slightly dampened spoon, flatten each mound into 2 ½-inch circles. Bake 9 to 10 minutes, until golden. Cool on sheets for an additional 10 minutes before transferring to racks to cool completely. Stored in an airtight container, cookies will keep fresh for 2 to 3 days (but probably won't last that long!)

Hidden Gem Cupcakes
Olive oil cooking spray
3 tbsp canola oil
2/3 cup light agave nectar
½ cup plus 1 tbsp unsweetened applesauce
1 tbsp flaxseeds, finely ground
1 tbsp pure vanilla extract
1 tbsp apple cider vinegar
2 cups light spelt flour, scooped and then leveled
1 tsp baking powder
1 tsp baking soda
½ tsp fine sea salt
1 cup berries (blueberries, raspberries, blackberries, chopped strawberries, or combination), fresh or frozen (do not thaw), divided, plus 12 raspberries for garnish
3 oz dark chocolate (70% cocoa), chopped
2 tbsp unsweetened almond or rice milk

Preheat oven to 350°F. Line 12 cups of a muffin tray with paper liners or mist with cooking spray.

In a small bowl, whisk together oil, agave nectar, applesauce, ¼ cup water, flaxseeds, vanilla, and vinegar. Set aside for at least 2 minutes while measuring dry ingredients.

In a large bowl, sift together flour, baking powder, baking soda, and salt. Stir briefly to combine. Pour wet mixture over dry mixture and stir to blend well.

Fill each muffin cup with about 1 tbsp batter, spreading to cover bottom and part way up the side of each cup. Place a heaping tsp of berries (about 4 to 5 berries) over the center of the batter, taking care not to let berries touch the sides of the cup. Top with another spoonful of batter, and gently spread batter to cover berries completely. Make sure to use all the batter, dividing evenly among 12 muffin cups.

Bake for 30 to 35 minutes, rotating tray about halfway through, until cupcakes are golden and a test inserted into the center comes out clean (it may be moist but shouldn't have any batter on it). Remove and allow to cool at room temperature for 5 minutes before removing cupcakes from tray to a cooling rack to cool completely.

Combine chocolate and milk in a large heatproof bowl set over a small pot of simmering water over low heat. Stir until chocolate melts and mixture is smooth and can be drizzled; add more milk if necessary to achieve desired texture.

Once cupcakes are cool, drizzle chocolate glaze in free-form lines across the top of each cupcake, then top with a raspberry. May be served immediately or stored at room temperature if serving later the same day. Cupcakes can also be stored, wrapped individually in plastic wrap, for up to 3 days in the refrigerator but should be enjoyed at room temperature.

Chocolate Sour Cream Cupcakes
1 cup unsweetened natural cocoa powder
1 ¼-cup Sucanat, divided

¼ cup whole-wheat pastry flour
¼ tsp kosher salt
¼ tsp baking soda
1 cup organic low-fat sour cream
1/3 cup plus 2 tsp skim milk, divided
1 tbsp olive oil
½ tsp pure vanilla extract
1 whole egg plus 2 egg whites
1 oz bittersweet chocolate, chopped, plus more for garnishment if desired

Preheat oven to 350°F. Line a 12 cup muffin pan with paper cupcake liners.

In a large mixing bowl, combine cocoa powder, 1 cup Sucanat, flour, salt and baking soda.

In a medium mixing bowl, whisk together sour cream, 1/3 cup milk, oil, vanilla, and whole egg.

Make a well in the center of the dry ingredients and pour in wet ingredients. Combine everything with a rubber spatula.

Add egg whites to a large clean, dry mixing bowl or the bowl of a stand mixer. Whip whites with hand beater or whisk attachment of stand mixer until they begin to get foamy. Add remaining ¼ cup Sucanat very gradually to whites. Continue whipping whites into medium-stiff peaks.

Fold whites into thirds into cake batter, gently but assertively with rubber spatula.

Fill each of the 12 cupcake liners ¾-full with batter. Tap bottom of filled muffin pan on countertop and transfer immediately to oven. Bake for 45 minutes or until a toothpick inserted in the center of a cupcake comes out clean.

Remove from oven and let cupcakes cool completely

When cupcakes are completely cool, combine chocolate and remaining 2 tsp milk in a microwave-safe bowl. Microwave on 50% power for 30 seconds. Stir until melted chocolate is completely smooth. Spread a thin layer on top of each cupcake. Sprinkle additional chocolate shavings on top, if desired.

Topping Take-Two:
Substitute ½ cup low-fat sour cream mixed with 1 tbsp honey for the chocolate glaze. Put a ½ tsp dollop on each cupcake and top with sliced strawberries.

Note: Adding monounsaturated-fat-rich olive oil, reducing the number of whole eggs and switching to Sucanat instead of white granulated sugar are just a few ways these cupcakes are a healthier choice for you!

Orange-Infused Chocolate-Almond Cake
Olive oil cooking spray
2 tbsp organic coconut oil, melted
2 tbsp smooth, unsalted almond butter
½ cup agave nectar
¼ cup prune puree (or all natural prune baby food)
2/3 cup orange juice, freshly squeezed
2tbsp flaxseeds, finely ground
2 tsp real vanilla extract
½ tsp balsamic vinegar
4 tsp orange zest, freshly grated
1 cup plus 2 tbsp light spelt flour, scooped then leveled
1/3 cup unsweetened dark cocoa powder, scooped and then leveled
¾ tsp baking soda

1 tsp baking powder
¼ tsp sea salt

Orange zest for garnish, grated (optional)
Blanched almonds for garnish (optional)

Glaze:
¾ cup orange juice, freshly squeezed
2 tbsp agave nectar

Cake:
Preheat oven to 350°F. Line the bottom of an 8 ½-inch springform pan with parchment paper; then mist paper and sides of pan with cooking spray.

In a small bowl, whisk together oil, almond butter and agave nectar until smooth. Add prune puree, juice, flaxseeds, vanilla, vinegar and zest, and mix well. Set aside, while you measure dry ingredients, for at least 2 minutes.

In a large bowl, sift together flour, cocoa, baking soda, baking powder and salt. Stir briefly to combine.

Pour wet mixture over dry one and stir well to blend. Pour into prepared pan and smooth the top.

Bake for 30 minutes then rotate pan 180° to ensure even baking and continue to bake for another 15 to 20 minutes, until cake springs back when pressed lightly in center. Remove from oven and allow to cool at room temperature while you prepare glaze.

Glaze:
Combine juice aand agave nectar in a small, heavy pot. Bring to boil over medium-high heat, then lower heat to simmer.

Allow mixture to bubble gently, stirring occasionally, until it reduces to about 1/3 cup, about 20 minutes. The mixture will turn deep golden and should coat a spoon.

Assembly:
Remove sides of pan from cooled cake. Slide a knife or metal spatula between parchment and bottom of the pan, then slip a serving plate into the gap and slide the cake onto it. Pour warm glaze over top of cake and gently spread toward the sides, allowing any excess to drip over the edges. Garnish with additional zest and almonds, if desired.

Serves 12

改善

Chapter 8: When to Eat and Why

W hat if the amount of food or the choices you put in your mouth didn't determine the size of your waistline as much as the TIMING of what you're eating?

Because of a series of insulin spikes in your blood stream and other scientific factors at play, it's true! You can determine your rate of weight loss based on WHEN you eat just as much as WHAT you eat!

Think about it: if you had a bowl of sugary cereal in the morning, your insulin production goes through the roof. We've covered that much already, right?

But what happens next? Remember how I told you that the insulin stays around for quite some time, eventually causing insulin resistance?

Turns out insulin, once produced, will remain in your body for FIVE HOURS. It just sits there, waiting for instruction or purpose. When it gets none, it begins to transform into fat.

Now, let's go back to that bowl of cereal you had this morning (in our example, anyway):

9:00am Bowl of Sugar Snacks
12:00pm Cheeseburger on a white bun with fries and a soda (yes, even diet – remember our talk on artificial sweeteners?)

You're already setting yourself up for a day of fat creation! Allowing only three hours between the time you ate the cereal to the time you consume all those fast-burning carbs, your insulin is still through the roof before you take your second bite of cheeseburger at lunch. Only 3 hours have passed since you ate breakfast and you still have an excess of insulin in your system!

So why is the "white bun" such an issue? It's a fast-burning carbohydrate. Same process as burning that sugary cereal this morning. You'll be hungry long before your insulin levels return to normal!

In fact, scientific research has found that, measured in calories, carbohydrates have 4 calories per gram (fats have 9 calories per gram! More on this in a few).

But all carbs are not created equal! We've talked briefly about slow and fast burning carbs. Slow burning carbs gently raise and lower your blood sugar, while the fast burning carbs shoot your sugar level off the charts faster than you can say, "Go!"

Why do we care? Because our blood sugar levels are closely connected with hunger, cravings, and the extent to which we store or burn fat.

We'll break this down into 2 stages, Beginner and Advanced.

The Beginner Stage is for those who are just starting out with the Kaizen method for weight loss and are still heavily relying on being guided through their eating and meals rather than the knowledge being 2nd nature yet.

Don't worry, beginners, we're gonna get there! Slow and steady wins the race and right now, you need to make sure you take it gradually to stay in the game!

The Advanced Stage is for those individuals who are comfortable with their food knowledge and can create a meal plan on the fly, regardless of what restaurant or grocery store they're in.

Beginner Stage

You're just starting out, so I want you to take it slow and easy. This is about making small changes, remember? Take your time and really make what you're doing a habit before you move on to the next step.

First up, the first meal of the day. Let's talk about breakfast. This meal is so important; I cannot even begin to tell you why it's so vital that you eat it!

So, step #1 – EAT BREAKFAST! This is the best way to start on your new eating plan. It literally means "break the fast" – meaning your body has gone all night without food and is in starvation mode. You gotta get something good in it and fast!

Now, if your excuse is, "I only have enough time to make a poptart and hit the road", I've got a solution for you:

The next time you're at the grocery store, pick up a few key items instead of those nasty poptarts to make breakfast an easy addition to your morning:

1. Ezekiel bread is best, but if you're pinching pennies (and who isn't), go for whole grain bread that has at least 2 grams of fiber per slice. Any less and chances are you're holding some poorly disguised white bread in drag!
2. Natural peanut butter (you'll know its natural if it only has 2 ingredients: peanuts and salt)

In the time it'd normally take you to pop your tart and hit the road, you'll be well on your way to eating a much healthier, weight-loss-focused breakfast!

The wheat in the bread will digest slower than breads made with white flour, and the peanut butter will give you a fuller feeling, high in protein and 'good fat'.

Remember, you'll wanna make breakfast a regular part of your day before moving on to the next step. We're slowly but surely ramping up your metabolism the way nature intended – one step at a time!

Step #2 – Chew your food slowly. If you're an emotional eater, you probably don't even realize that you've eaten anything. The food magically vanishes off your plate.

If you're feeling guilty about eating, you might not even taste the food. You go into "robot mode" and your hand mechanically goes from the plate to your mouth without feeling or enjoying what's in it.

I've done it more times than I can count! The worse I believe the food to be for me, the faster I eat it. This one took me quite a while to conquer with steady, deliberate movements when I eat.

You see, before you can begin to think about keeping the weight off, you've got to develop a healthier relationship with your food.

Food isn't what made you overweight. You did by the eating and lifestyle choices that you made. Likewise, food isn't going to make you thinner. You are by the eating and lifestyle choices that you're making now.

Between each bite of food, put your fork down, chew the food in your mouth and really NOTICE how it tastes. You may be tasting food that you've eaten for years – for the first time!

Do not put another bite of food in your mouth until the food that's currently occupying that space has been swallowed.

If you're really struggling with this one (this was the hardest one for me to overcome), set a timer at each meal and make it a point to let the timer go off before you've finished with your meal. So if you set the timer for 20 minutes (in the beginning, maybe 5 minutes if you're anything like I was), make certain you don't finish eating until after the 20 minutes have elapsed, chewing slowly and deliberately. Take your time and re-learn that food isn't the enemy. ***And it never will be again.***

Step #3 - Eat 5-6 times a day. This one'll take some getting use to, to be sure! Start off just having a small snack a few hours after breakfast.

If you work a 9-5, this may mean taking a piece of fruit with you to work in the mornings.

If you're a full-time parent, this could be having a snack with your kids (they're usually hungry about this time). But instead of cookies and treats, have some fruit slices, a handful of 10 almonds, or something a bit healthier.

As you become use to eating your mid-morning snack, you'll notice your fatigue in the afternoons begin to wane. Because you're giving your body the fuel it needs to survive (and your metabolism is going up, up, up!) you aren't as fatigued in the afternoon.

Now its time to add the next mini-meal to your day. Mid-afternoon. Opt for something higher in protein and lower in carbohydrates to keep you from spiking that insulin we talked about earlier. Think protein shake (recipe in the previous chapter), maybe a 2oz piece of grilled or baked chicken.

If you find yourself trying too hard to get in your afternoon snack, scale it back and just try to have a handful of nuts. Don't overthink this. You wanna make it habit first.

Step #4 – Water. Drink it. Chances are, you aren't drinking as much water as you should be. By a long shot. In fact, if I cut you and you bleed diet cola, we have a problem.

So I want you to get a water bottle. Put it somewhere you'll see it often. On your desk. In the nursery. Wherever. Your goal is to drink that bottle today. Don't let your head hit the pillow without finishing that one single bottle of water.

Your goal will eventually be to have drank 8-10 glasses of H2O daily. But you gotta walk it up. You aren't gonna stop drinking diet sodas overnight and for me to tell you that it must be done will only drive you to want them more.

Once you've gotten use to having your one bottle of water a day, up it to 2. Then 3. Eventually, use your diet drink as a reward for drinking the amount of water your body needs in a day.

When you're drinking 3-4 bottles of water a day, I want you to look at your body in the mirror. In the way your clothes fit.

Often times, your body has been trying to "make due" with the garbage you've been giving it and therefore has been running at minimum efficiency. Now that you're giving it water regularly, a few things are happening:

1. You're in the bathroom more regularly (oh, don't get embarrassed. There's an entire chapter on fiber and pooh later in the book.) and its...easier!
2. You're losing more weight than you expected (maybe not on the scale. But in the way your clothes fit and on the tape measure – where it counts!)
3. You feel better. Constant aches in your joints are going away. Hello – it's because you've been lubricating these joints with the right kind of liquid. Water is a true miracle worker when it comes to health and your body!Notice I didn't say stop drinking sodas or coffee. We both know you aren't gonna do it at first. I need you to recognize on your own that these extras do your body no good and should be eventually eliminated.

Master these 4 stages before you even think about moving on to the Advanced Stage. You need these basic principles to be

HABIT, an EVERYDAY OCCURANCE, and failing to get these down could spell disaster later on.

In the Advanced Stage, we'll take a look at how much you should be eating, then we'll divvy it up into the meals you'll have in a day!

> If you find that you've got difficulty getting rid of certain drinks, check out the "Overcoming Cravings" chapter in the book, or leave your name and email address on my blog at www.WhatIfYOUWereThin.com and get my "107 Secrets to Overcoming Temptation" series.

Advanced Stage

Alright guys, time to crank your nutrition up a notch! You've gotten use to throwing out the first bite, to eating smaller portions, to passing a McArches without veering for the drive thru, but now we gotta take your eating plan to the next level!

I will warn you, this is gonna require some math on your part!

I took Math 100 twice in college (that's the most basic, Math-for-Dummies level you can take and I took it twice because I hate math so much and never went to class). Needless to say, this is really the only portion of the book that'll have this many formulas and equations in it!

First, we'll determine the number of calories you need to consume in a day (note the different equation for men and women). To do this, we need to convert your weight from pounds to kilograms and your height from inches to centimeters:

Take your current weight in pounds, divide it by 2.2, and that's your weight in kilograms. For example, a 150pound woman would look like this:

150/ 2.2 = 16.181kg

Next, the height conversion. Take your height in inches, and multiply it by 2.54 to find your height in centimeters. Our 150 pound woman is 5'5", that's 60 inches total. She'd look like this:

60 x 2.54 = 152.4cm

Now, let's find how many calories you must consume in a day just to stay alive:

Male: 66.5+ (13.75 x W) + (5.003 x H) − (6.775 x A)
Female: 65.1+ (9.563 x W) + (1.850 x H) − (4.676 x A)

W = actual weight in kg
H = actual height in cm
A = age in years

This gives you the amount of calories you need just to live. That doesn't include the burning of calories during your workout, or tell you how much to eat at each meal! There's a little bit more math to go! Stay with me!

We're going to divide up the allotted calories in your day into the three main sections we'll be tracking: protein, carbohydrates, and fat.

We're going by the 40/40/20 rule, which means 40% of your calories will come from protein, 40% of your calories will come from carbohydrates, and 20% of your calories will come from fat. This ensures you'll have a proper balance of everything your body needs to shed the weight (and keep it off!)

So, if your daily caloric intake (which we got from that slightly painful formula above) is 1500, you'd divide 1500 by .4 to find how much protein and carbohydrates you'll eat in a day. You'll divide the same 1500 calories by .2 to find out how much fat you'll eat in a day:

1500/.4= 600 calories of your daily intake will be protein
1500/.4= 600 calories of your daily intake will be carbohydrates
1500/.2= 300 calories of your daily intake will be from fat

(Make certain you do these calculations with the actual numbers you came up with earlier!)

Now, just a little more math, and the pain will be over with! ☺

There are 4 calories per gram of both carbohydrates and protein. So we'll divide the number of calories you'll take in today from protein by 4 to see how many grams of protein you'll need to eat:

For our example above, that's 600 (calories) divided by 4 (calories per gram of protein) = 150 grams of protein per day.

The same will hold true for carbohydrates, meaning you'll do the same calculation and have 150 grams of carbohydrates per day.

Finally, there's fat. This stuff has 9 calories per gram of fat, so naturally, you'll have less fat in your diet than you will protein or carbs, right?

300 (the number of calories from fat in our example above) divided by 9 (calories per gram of fat) = 33.33 grams of fat per day

So now we know how much to eat in order to be fit, let's look at WHEN to eat, rather than HOW MUCH:

It's the 'When' More Than the 'What'

This is kinda the fun part of this program because you get to play around with your meal plan and really make it your own.

Just like you wouldn't pick up a weight and follow what works for the bodybuilder working out next to you, your meal plan should be customized to what works best for YOU.

You'll wanna eat most of your quick burning carbs as early in the day as possible, to allow your insulin level to have enough time to balance itself out the rest of the day.

Look back at the formula you used earlier to calculate the amount of fat, protein, and carbs you'll need in a day and have at least half of the carbs and fat you're allotted by lunch.

Remember how I told you that insulin stays in your body for 5 hours, looking for something to do before it turns into fat? By eating most of your carbs and fat in the first half of the day, you're doing several things for your body!

1. You're eliminating that tired feeling after lunch. It's a thing of the past! Your body is gonna draw on the storage of carbohydrates you've just given it in the first 3 meals of your day for energy.

2. As the day turns into evening, you'll find it easier to fall asleep too! You aren't hopped up on sugar and spiking your insulin to make it difficult to slow your body down in preparation for bedtime! Imagine, waking up refreshed tomorrow and ready for a new day all because you've eaten well the night before!

Look, I'm not expecting you to be perfect every single day. Some days you'll have more of one thing or another than you're supposed to. On occasion, you might fall off the wagon altogether.

This isn't an excuse to 'cheat' or eat something you shouldn't. You're human and it happens. Just try to stick to the amounts you calculated for yourself and do the best you can. The results will prove to be worth the effort, I promise!

To Sum It Up
1. "When" to eat is just as important as "what" to eat!
2. If you're in the Beginner Stage, eat breakfast to begin your kaizen transformation. It jumpstarts your metabolism and increases your energy for the day!
3. Chew your food slowly and enjoy what you're eating. Food is no longer the enemy!
4. Eat 5-6 meals a day to rev up your metabolism and keep from binging when you get hungry.
5. Drink more water. You'll feel fuller, have an easier time in the bathroom, and your skin will even look better!
6. As you advance, eat your starchy carbs towards the beginning of the day to keep your insulin levels down and your energy up, up, up!

Chapter 9: How to Overcome Cravings

I know you'd like to think that since you purchased this book that all of your cravings will be a thing of the past.

Wrong.

I still have cravings. I still have trouble walking past the cookie aisle at the grocery store and not wanting to have one of each.

But here's where a word will come into play that I haven't used in this book until now...Willpower. I know, not a fun word to read, even less fun to implement. But the fact of the matter is that you're gonna have to start walking away from the sweets, the salties, the cravings you have late at night.

The good news is that I'm gonna give you a few tried and true tips to overcoming your cravings once and for all.

Now, if you're just starting out, remember, the name of the game is KAIZEN – good change (in little steps).

Step 1 – Indulge Yourself!
The next time you're dying for a candybar, have it. Just throw out the first bite. Go ahead! I said you can eat the candybar, but not the first bite.

I can't take credit for this idea. It came from Dr. Robert Maurer, PhD. He applies the kaizen method to every single aspect of your life in his book "One Small Step Can Change Your Life" (a great book. I highly recommend it!)

Throwing out the first bite is gonna do something to you psychologically. (Bear with me, I'm goin' deep!) Because you didn't eat the WHOLE candybar, you don't trigger that guilt response that comes after eating something you know to be 'bad' for you.

But it also isn't enough to give you permission to have a 2nd one.

In addition, the stigma of throwing away perfectly good food may eventually be enough of a burden that you would rather do without the candybar than to throw away food (remember mom telling you about the starving children around the world?)

Take time to throw out the first bite until it becomes 2nd nature to you. This could take a week, 3 weeks, or even a month or two – but if you aren't prepared to do what's necessary to lose the weight, taking the next step will only result in failure and we don't want that!

Step 2 – No Substitutions!

This is one time I'm not gonna suggest an apples-to-apples comparison.

If you're ready to move to the next step, after throwing out the first bite, we're gonna have to talk substitution.

That means, if you want something sweet, find something other than your normal go-to-candy.

Want chocolate? Have some watermelon.
Want sour candy? Try an apple.
Want something sweet? Have a slice of pineapple.

But this goes for more than just candy!

Want salty chips? Have some sweet potato fries.
Want something savory? Fill yourself up with some oatmeal.

No doubt, you're starting to get bummed. I know. But there's a method to this madness.

Remember that talk we had earlier about artificial sweeteners? They do more than just give you access to some pretty unhealthy chemicals.

They also trick your mind into thinking that you're having the thing you want and that it's ok. But it's NOT!

I know some folks who've been on a carbohydrate-free diet for years and have literally substituted their love of 'all things sugar' for the sugar-free kind. You have a candybar? They have the sugar-free candybar. You have a piece of gum? They have sugar-free gum. You have a scoop of ice cream? They have the ENTIRE CONTAINER of sugar-free ice cream.

They claim to not be tempted by sugary sweets..because they're getting the sugar-free version.

But the answer to wanting sugar isn't to substitute it for something that'll only kill you in a different way! It's like saying, "I don't want to die from cancer, so I'm gonna give myself a heart attack instead." It just doesn't make sense!

You want to break your mind of these cravings and the only way to do it is to let your mind know that it's **not** ok to eat these types of sweets and salty indulgences.

Not to mention the fact that, just because it says "Sugar Free" on the container, it doesn't mean there's no calories or fat! Often times, in order to make something still palatable, the manufacturers must add fat to a sugar-free product to get people to buy it.

And guess what the body likes to do with fat? STORE IT ON YOUR BUTT!

Bottom line – no sugar-free or fat-free substitutes. Find a clean alternative like fruit, nuts, or veggies to nosh on until the craving passes.

Step 3 – The Final Straw!
The last step is the easiest and the hardest all at the same time.

Simply don't have it in the house.

I don't care how much your family enjoys Tons o' Chips cookies. They don't need them and neither do you!

It's not about making sure the kids or the spouse has what they love to eat anymore. This is a lifestyle change and they need to recognize that you'll eat this way forever. Not just for the next month or 12 weeks.

If you can't stop eating it, then stop buying it.

If the kids beg for stuff when you're at the grocery store, stop taking them with you…or just say no.

Your eating from here on out needs to eventually become NON-Negotiable. You wanna lose weight? You gotta step your game up and really make certain you're watching what you put in your mouth.

You've done the "throw out the first bite" thing. You've substituted what you crave for something healthier. But if you can't keep from putting the entire pan of brownies in your face like I use to, then you gotta stop bringing it home.

For me, the guilt of using gasoline and wear and tear on the car just to go get something I knew I shouldn't have was enough to keep me from driving to get it.

Here's some other Craving Busters you can use:

1. Have 16oz of water before you eat anything. Many times, we're actually dehydrated and it's hard to tell the difference between dehydration and hunger.
2. Buy smaller plates. Your smaller portions look bigger and fool your mind into thinking your eating more than you are!
3. Take 2 laps around your house or apartment complex before indulging. If the craving is still there, eat in moderation.
4. Tell yourself you can wait 30 minutes before giving in. Then find something else to do with your hands. You'll

either forget the craving or discover you don't want it as bad as you thought you did!

5. Get a hobby. Preferably something outside of the kitchen that will keep your hands busy.
6. Stay away from gum. The chewing action plus the fruity smell of the gum often triggers a response in our brain to make us want to eat – the exact opposite of why you got the gum in the first place!
7. Drink 10 eight ounce glasses of water throughout the day. The water makes you feel fuller and you don't notice the hunger pangs as often.
8. Eat small meals every 2-3 hours to keep from getting hungry.

The point here is to make certain your body knows that you're on the path to good health and don't want to be derailed by cravings.

Legally Cheating

If you find yourself giving in every once in a while – don't panic. It's actually ok to give yourself a "cheat meal" once a week!

This allows you to focus your energy on saving up for that one blessed day when you can have anything you want (yes, anything! Ice cream, chocolate, sweet and sour chicken with fried rice, anything!) rather than the cycle you've had until now.

Cycle? Oh, you know. The craving strikes, you "cheat" on your diet. You feel guilty, beat yourself up mentally, then figure since you've already cheated, why not go back for more? Then the whole plan is out the window and you'll start again on Monday because who starts a diet in the middle of the week?

Well now, you can set a day that allows you to have one meal of anything you want!

Pancakes and sausage? Go for it.
Double quarter pound cheeseburger and fries? Sure.
Uber-sized Milkshake? Of course.

Just make sure it's *one meal* and not the whole day. (Incidentally, if you do the whole day, you'll notice it around 1-2pm. The sluggishness, the lethargy. You'll wonder how you ever ate like that all the time and then vow never to do that to yourself again.)

Not only does this do great things for you psychologically, but it also tricks your metabolism!

Your body says, "Hey, look at all this great stuff we've gotten during this meal! We don't need to hold on to every single calorie since there'll be more later on!" Sometimes, I'd find that I lost weight the day after a cheat meal (this isn't necessarily typical, but is fun when it happens!)

Plan your whole week around your "cheat meal" and really make it something you'll enjoy. Don't worry about going 'whole hog', though. Remember, you get another one in just one more week, so you can plan what you'll have for that one and have something to look forward to!

Just remember that you're human and allow yourself a little wiggle room. You've worked hard during those 6 days to eat right and do well. Now reward yourself with a meal of your choice!

To Sum It Up

1. Indulge yourself – But throw out the first bite!
2. No substitutions for your sugary favs with it's sugar-free

alternative. Don't let your mind think it's ok to still eat garbage!

3. If you can't control yourself, then don't bring it home. If you know you'll eat it all in one sitting, then don't buy it at all.

4. Drink water, buy smaller plates, eat smaller meals more often, and stay away from gum to reduce cravings!

5. Cheating is ok on your "cheat meal day". One meal, once a week. No more. No less!

改善

Chapter 10: Safe Eating List

emember how we talked about good/bad fats, slow/fast burning carbs, etc? Wonder how you were gonna keep em all straight?

Here's your guide to choosing what you'll eat in a day. Refer back to Chapter 8 on when to eat and why to fit what you're going to eat into your daily schedule.

Protein Choices:

All fish and shellfish
Lean beef
Venison
Turkey breast or leg (skinless)
Rabbit
Chicken breast or leg (skinless)

Minced beef
Lean pork
Duck breast (skinless)
Veal
Lamb
Ham
Eggs (3 whole or 5 whites)
Cottage cheese

Protein powder

Low fat cheese (less than 10% fat)

Ricotta cheese

Low or fat-free Greek yogurt

*Beware the cheeses. They are great sources of protein but contain a lot of saturated fat. Always eat a matchbox sized portion of cheese when in doubt.

Carbohydrate Choices:

Alfalfa sprouts
Arugula
Bamboo shoots
Bok choy
Broccoli
Cabbage
Carrots
Cauliflower
Celery
Chicory
Cucumber
Endive
Fennel
Lettuce
Mushrooms
Onions
Peas
Peppers
Radishes
Spinach
Tomatoes

Water chestnuts
Watercress
Artichokes
Asparagus
Beans
Beets
Brussels sprouts
Chickpeas
Eggplant
Green beans
Hummus
Lentils (all kinds)
Okra
Pumpkin
Spinach
Zucchini
Apples
Apricots

Blackberries
Black currants
Blueberries
Cherries
Grapefruit
Grapes
Kiwi fruit
Lemons/Limes
Melons
Nectarines
Oranges
Peaches
Pears
Fresh Pineapple
Plums
Red currants
Strawberries
Tangerines
Watermelon

*Keep your fruit portions to a minimum each day due to the amount of fructose (the sugar contained in fruit).

Fat Choices:

Almonds

Cashew nuts

Hazelnuts

Avocado

Brazil nuts

Canola or avocado oil
(cold-pressed)

Flaxseed

Extra virgin olive oil

Macadamia nuts

Natural peanut butter

Peanuts

Pistachios

Pine nuts

Pumpkin seeds

Sunflower seeds

Walnuts

Vinaigrette

Sesame paste (tahini)

Clarified butter, or ghee

Mayonnaise

Sesame oil

*Keep an eye on the amount of Saturated Fat you're eating when choosing what to dine on! If possible, keep the amount of saturated fat you eat to 0 or as close to it as possible. Some meats will naturally have a small amount of saturated fat, but when reading your nutrition label – look for mono or polyunsaturated fats for your best options!

Remember, we figured out how much of each choice (protein, carbohydrates, fat) you can have earlier in the book, so refer back to Chapter 8 if you've got questions on the amount of each you can have!

To Sum It Up
1. Matchbox-sized cheese portions keep the fat content to a minimum.
2. Eat as much of the carbs as you want (but keep your fruit intake to a minimum – no more than 5oz at a meal)!
3. Read the recommended portion size on the side of the nutrition label to ensure you're eating the right amount!

改善

Chapter 11: Meal Planning Calendar

ow that you've figured out how much you should eat in a day, the types of foods you can be looking for, and what to stay away from (even how to bust cravings) – it's time to put what you've learned into practice!

Here's a sample page from my own food journal that may offer some insight into how you should be eating:

Food	Calories	Protein	Carbs	Fat
Breakfast (7am)				
1 cup grits	150	8.4	23.5	2.4
16oz. coffee	5	1	0	0
1 cup milk	147	7.9	12.9	8.1
TOTAL	**297**	**17.3**	**36.4**	**10.5**
Mid-morning snack (10am)				
5oz watermelon	43	.9	10.8	.3

12 almonds	69	2.6	2.4	6.1
TOTAL	**112**	**3.5**	**13.2**	**6.4**
Lunch (noon)				
4oz chicken	188	35.2	0	4
10 asparagus spears	32	3.5	6.2	.2
6oz beans	244	15.4	44.6	1.2
2Tbsp BBQ sauce	35	0	8	1
TOTAL	**499**	**54.1**	**58.8**	**6.2**
Post-workout shake (3pm)				
30g protein powder	130	23	3	2
8oz water	0	0	0	0
TOTAL	**130**	**23**	**3**	**2**
Dinner (5pm)				
2oz chicken	94	17.6	0	2
1cup salad	17	1.3	3.3	.1
2Tbsp fat free balsamic vinaigrette dressing	35	0	8	0
TOTAL	**146**	**18.9**	**11.3**	**2.1**
Daily Total	**1184**	**116.8**	**122.7**	**27.2**
Daily Allowance	**1193**	**119**	**119**	**26.5**
Results	**-8**	**-2.2**	**+3.7**	**+.7**

You'll note that my breakfast alone had almost half my fat for the day! After lunch, my carb and fat counts drop way down (I only ate 14.3g carbs and 4.1g fat), allowing me to drastically reduce my insulin levels by bedtime.

You'll also note that I ate very well throughout the day. I didn't starve, was never hungry, and even went a few grams over on some of my "allowance".

So here's what you do:

1. Go to your local Everything-Mart and pick up a spiral notebook (or use Microsoft Excel on your computer).
2. Create columns as I have above for your food, calories, carbs, protein, and fat.
3. Track each day every single morsel that you put in your mouth (yes, everything).
4. Compare this against the formula we created earlier where you figured out your daily allowance of food.

Keep track of your eating for at least 4 weeks. I want at least 3 weekends in your food journal so you can see if you go off-track, if you're better at sticking to the plan on specific days, etc.

Worst case scenario, I included my own nutrition tracker worksheet in the Worksheets section of this book for you to print and use on your own. You've got no excuse for great nutrition!

Additional Tips and Tricks

Plan out your entire weeks' worth of eating and use that as your grocery list. Then, DO NOT BUY anything if it isn't on your list! This eliminates the craving to buy that one thing you can't resist (mine's anything chocolate).

Eat before you go grocery shopping to keep the impulse buying at bay. (They stick the chocolate bars by the register for a reason, you know!)

Stick to the outer walls of the grocery store. This is where most of the freshest ingredients will be and that's what you want. Remember, you should be able to grow it, pick it, or get it lean from the butcher. Otherwise, you don't really want it.

A Word on Salads

You're going to kaizen your way into eating a lot more fresh fruits and vegetables. Even eating more salads!

Never let your salad get boring. You aren't restricted to just lettuce and tomato. There are a plethora of other salad-greens available to you!

Spinach
Bok choy
Napa cabbage

Each have their own flavor and texture that can really make a salad a new experience. Don't be afraid to try a new vegetable or fruit the next time you're in the grocery store. You never know what green leaf you'll fall in love with!

To Sum It Up:

1. Once you're advanced enough to track your caloric intake, get a notebook and write down everything you put in your mouth to see just how much you've "really" been eating!
2. Eat before you go grocery shopping to avoid unnecessary purchases.
3. Keep your salads interesting by varying the types of ingredients you choose!

Now – on to Kaizen Fitness!

Part II - Kaizen Fitness

改善

Chapter 12: Getting Started

*I*f someone had tried to talk to me about exercise when I first started my own weight loss journey 70+ pounds ago – all I envisioned were days of sweating, waiting to die, and feeling so sore afterwards that I didn't want to get out of bed.

And at the time, I was right! Because I hadn't been properly educated on fitness and the role of nutrition in weight loss, I expected that the harder I worked out, the more weight I'd lose.

But you've already got a leg up on where I was because I'm teaching you that a fantastic body is made in the kitchen and you're gonna sculpt that body with exercise. Not the other way 'round!

So on the following pages are 3 different Kaizen workouts that you can choose from in order to begin a proper workout regimine without fear of reprocussions from co-workers, your spouse, or anyone else (because in most of these cases, no one will be able to tell that you're working out!

Do the workout of your choice for at least 21 days (that's when it becomes a "habit" in the mind).

Choose the workout that either appeals to you most or will fit best into your daily life:

The Commercial Break Program: This one's for the on-your-feeters (mostly in the service industry) who are just too tired to when they get home from work to think about exercise OR who get up early enough as it is and can't fathom setting the alarm clock an hour earlier just to workout.

The 4 Minute Workout: This one's for parents who's time is not their own. Feel like you live to bus your kids to soccer practice (you can do the exercises in your car) or can't wait til naptime to actually get something done in the day? This one's for you!

Easy Office Fitness: This one's for the desk-jobbers who spend their day in a cubicle or behind a desk. You'll start out in 4 minute increments that you can do on break, during your work day, or anytime you can fit them in!

Remember, just choose one workout program and work through it for the 21 days. Each one starts you out SLOWLY to build the habit.

Now that you've got the basic overview, let's get to the nitty gritty!

Chapter 13: The Commercial Break Program

*I*f you've ever come home from spending the day on your feet, this is your program! You're exhausted and barely have enough energy to kick off your shoes to get to the couch and crash. Been there, done that!

So with this program, you'll wanna pay special attention to the length of your workout as well as the particular exercise you're doing.

What you'll need to get started: yourself. Nothing else. (In exercise #4 you'll need a phone book or basketball, but it'll be something you've already got in your house and don't need to purchase anything!)

To do the Commercial Break Program (the Kaizen way), you'll start exercising with *just one commercial* during your favorite show. Pick just one commercial and stand up. It's only for 30 seconds (and you can do 30 seconds, right?) Then you're done. Don't even think about exercise for the rest of the day. You did it!

Now, because this is Kaizen, you'll want to eventually move up the length of your workout to two commercials, then three and so on until you can exercise during the entire break. But only move up when you feel you're ready (aka when the exercise has gotten too easy to do during the one commercial). This could take a week, maybe longer.

But for now, let's just start with one exercise movement, one commercial. Do this every night for 21 days. Hey, it's only 30 seconds!

You'll notice during the description of the exercise moves below that they get progressively harder as you move through them. They're designed to challenge your body without being overwhelming or painful.

As always, you should consult your doctor before beginning any exercise regime and get his go-ahead before continuing.

Exercise #1: March in place. Simply lift your left knee up as high as you can, then put it back down on the ground and repeat on the right side.

Exercise #2: Shoulder touches. Stand up straight with your shoulders back. Touch your fingertips to the tops of your shoulders, keeping your elbows pointed away from your body. Inhale as you raise your arms to the ceiling. Exhale as you bring your fingertips back down to touch the tops of your shoulders. Repeat.

Exercise #3: Toe touches. Stand up straight with your shoulders back. Keeping a soft bend in your knees and a flat back, exhale as you reach down to touch your toes. Go as far as you can to feel tension in the backs of your legs, but not pain. Inhale to stand back up. Repeat.

Note: If you have issues with blood pressure, be mindful when doing this exercise and go slowly to avoid light-headedness. If you do feel light-headed, go slower or sit down and wait for the next commercial.

Exercise #4: Adductor squeeze. Grab a phone book, a thick text book, or a basketball (or at the very least, a towel to put between your knees). This is the only exercise you'll need "equipment" for. Place your object between your knees. Stand up straight and tall. Use your knees and adductor muscles (the parts of your thighs that sometimes rub together when you walk) to squeeze the object between your knees for one second (as in "one-one thousand, two-one thousand"-type counting). Relax. Repeat.

Exercise #5: Warrior 1. Stand with your feet wide apart. Not enough to be uncomfortable like you're doing the splits. But wide enough that a grown adult could crawl through your legs. Turn your left toe 90 degrees away from your body. Turn your right heel 35 degrees away from your body. Turn your torso to the left, in line with your left foot. While simultaneously inhaling as much air as you can, bend your left knee to as close of a 90 degree, keeping your back leg straight. Raise your arms above your head and touch the palms of your hands together with your elbows straight. Hold this position for 15 seconds and then repeat on the other side. Holding this position, once on each side, will take up the entire commercial you're working through.

Exercise #6: Side lunge. Stand with your feet wide apart. (As in Warrior 1.) While simultaneously pushing your rear towards the wall behind you, bend your left knee and move your body to the left. Keep your right leg and your back straight. You can keep your hands on your hips, hold them out in front of you, or slightly place them on your left thigh for support (but don't lean!) Hold this position for 2 full seconds. Return to your standing position. Repeat on the right side.

Only move up to the next exercise when you feel you're ready. Take your time and enjoy getting fit! You deserve it!

When you're ready to advance to more difficult workouts, even including weights, log onto my Members-Only site at www.WhatIfYOUWereThin.com to find an entire year's worth of workouts you can use!

Chapter 14: The 4 Minute Workout

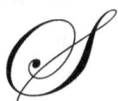

Shhhh! The kids are finally down for a nap! You've actually got some time (dare you think it!) to...yourself! What do you do first? Clean the house? Fold laundry? NO!

It's time to take care of YOU! You can't properly take care of anyone else if you aren't looking out for your own health and wellbeing.

The laundry is not going to self-destruct if you don't fold it right this second. The cleaning isn't going to get so overwhelming that you can't do it later.

Right now, you've got 4 solid minutes to do something to strengthen your body and make yourself a better parent (and probably spouse)!

The 4 Minute Workout is exactly what you need! But every second counts in this workout, so I've combined several movements to work different muscles at the same time, allowing you to burn maximum calories while getting this over with as fast as possible!

So **each move is going to be just 30 seconds long**. And before you know it – 4 minutes have passed and you can go about your day knowing you've done great things for your health…and your family! But first, we gotta get you warmed up!

Step 1: March in place for 30 seconds. Nothing too fast or strenuous. Just get the blood flowing.

Step 2: Jumping Jacks. Begin standing with your feet together and arms at your sides. As you jump into the air, bring your feet slightly wider than shoulder width apart. At the same time, bring your arms straight above your head and clap your hands together. Jump again and return to your starting position. Repeat for the duration of the commercial.

Step 3: Squat and Press. You can grab a couple of cans from the cupboard if you want, or do this empty handed if you're just starting out.

Stand with your feet approximately hip distance apart with your arms bent at a 90 degree angle. Keep your abs tight! You're gonna be using your core!

Now, imagine a chair behind you. Pretend to sit in the chair by pushing your rear towards the wall behind you while bending your knees. During the entire movement, keep your knees in the same place, making sure they don't roll in as you "sit". Be certain to keep your knees behind your toes! Your back should be straight, shoulders back, and if I were standing in front of you, I should have a clear view of your chest. Inhale as you sit and hold that position for 2 seconds, exhaling as you return to a standing position and pressing your arms over your head with a straight elbow. Repeat.

Step 4: Forward Lunge with a Hammer Curl. You can also use some cans from the cupboard on this one, or do it empty handed if you're just starting out.

Place your left foot directly in front of you so that your feet are approximately 2 feet apart. With your hands at your sides, inhale as you bend your knees so that they are both at a 90 degree angle. At the same time, bend your elbows and raise your hands to your shoulders, keeping your elbows by your side. Squeeze your biceps as you raise your hands. Your back knee should hover just above the ground without actually touching the ground. Once again, keep your back straight, eyes looking straight ahead, and do not let your front knee go over your front toe. Your back toes will remain on the ground while the heel will come up slightly as you bend your knee. Exhale as you come up and return your hands to your sides.

The farther apart your feet, the more emphasis you place on your rear.

The closer your feet are together, the more emphasis you place on your quadriceps (upper thigh muscles).

Step 5: Anterior raise with a side lunge. Stand with your feet wide apart. While simultaneously pushing your rear towards the wall behind you, bend your left knee and move your body to the left. Keep your right leg and your back straight. With straight elbows, raise your arms in front of you to shoulder length as you lunge, concentrating on your shoulder muscles.

Hold this position for 2 full seconds. Return to your standing position, lowering your arms back to your sides. Repeat on the right side.

Step 6: Plank. You won't move an inch, but will be working virtually every muscle in your body! Get onto the floor, lying on your stomach. With a flat back and strong abs, raise yourself off the floor until only your elbows, forearms, hands, and toes are supporting you. Keep your ears, shoulders, hips, knees and ankles in a straight line. You will hold this move for the full 30 seconds.

Note: if you're just starting out and cannot hold for the full 30 seconds, rather than giving up, drop down onto your knees for a few seconds to catch your breath. Then return to the full plank position. The results are soooo worth it!

Now you're ready to tackle the day and have more energy to get it all done. You're a superhero!

Want something more challenging? Log onto my Members-Only site at www.WhatIfYOUWereThin.com to find an entire year's worth of workouts you can use!

Chapter 15: Easy Office Fitness

Another day at the office, huh? No time to workout. You get up before the sun. You get home in time to crash on the couch. Who has time to exercise?

You do, now! And you can do it without leaving your desk, without alerting your co-workers to the fact that you're getting fit, and without going to an embarrassing gym!

In fact, I've given some of these exercise moves names that you can use as excuses if someone happens to walk by your desk while you're doing them!

There's no time limit on these moves, but you'll see best results from doing each one for at least 30 seconds. There's a worksheet at the end of this book to keep track of your results!

I'm concentrating on a new idea: (*This works your arm and chest muscles!*) Clasp your hands together in front of your chest, as if arm wrestling your own hand. Keep your elbows straight out to your sides. Pressing the palms of your hands together, contract your chest muscles as you press. Hold for 1 second, relax. Repeat.

Nothing, why?: (*This works your back and shoulder muscles!*) Keeping your elbows out to your sides, clasp your fingers together and use your back and shoulders to try and "pull" your fingers apart. Pull straight out to the side and don't let your fingers come apart! Hold for 1 second, relax. Repeat.

Goofing off: (*This works your abs!*) Sit on the edge of your chair with your hands griping either side of the chair, or resting on each side of your buttocks where possible, feet off the floor. Inhale and bring your knees to your chest while rounding the back at the same time. Return to the initial position while exhaling, and begin again.

Just stretching my legs: (*This works your behind, hamstrings, and quadriceps!*) Position your feet about shoulder width apart while sitting in your chair. Keep your head and back straight. Exhale and stand up without using any support from the chair. Slowly inhale, pushing your hips back, allowing your knees to bend naturally and your torso to lean forward. When you go to sit back down, do not let your behind touch the chair. Come down as far as you can, then stand back up. Repeat.

No fake reasoning needed: (*This works the inside of your thighs!*) No one will be able to see you doing this one! Grab a phone book, a text book, or a basketball (or at the very least, a towel to put between your knees). This is the only exercise you'll need "equipment" for. Place your object between your knees. Sit up straight and tall. Scoot your chair close to your desk so no one can see you. Use your knees and adductor muscles (the parts of your thighs that rub together when you walk) to squeeze the object between your knees for one second (as in "one-one thousand"-type counting). Relax. Repeat.

Another invisible move: (*This one works your calf muscles!*) Start by sitting in your office chair. Find a heavy encyclopedia, textbook, phone book, or otherwise "heavy" object and place it in your lap. If you're just starting out, no object may be necessary in the beginning. Begin to exhale, activate the core, and extend the ankles to life the knees and the weight. Press up as far as possible, keeping the ankles from rolling out and keeping the weight over the balls of the feet. Continue to contract the core and trunk muscles. Hold, then slowly inhale and allow the legs to lower down to the starting position while maintaining proper posture and ankle positioning.

Extra Office Fitness:

- Take the stairs instead of the elevator.
- Park at the back of the parking lot and walk to your office door.
- Replace your chair at work with a stability ball.
- Walk for half of your lunch hour. Then eat.
- Perform 'wall pushups' in a conference room or bathroom stall.

There are Advanced Easy Office Fitness moves available when you log on to the Members-Only section at www.WhatIfYOUWereThin.com!

Chapter 16: When You're Ready to Join a Gym

A t this point, you've been doing one of the workouts long enough that you're paying more attention to it than the tv show you were watching, lose track of when the commercial is over because you're so into it, or are ready for more of a challenge.

It's time to hit the gym!

I'll admit, I enjoyed doing it all on my own at first, but WOW! What a difference a gym can make! In fact, joining a gym helped me break through a plateau I'd been on and lead me to lose the last 7 pounds to my goal weight!

Just as with choosing a spouse, you're gonna want to "date" your gym. There are specific qualities you need to look for before you even go on your first "date" and then when you say "I do", you gotta make sure you really want to commit!

Here are a few things to keep in mind when looking for a gym:

Price
I've spoken before on teleseminars and other events - but there's a lot to be said for price vs. cost. They're not the same thing.

When I first started looking for a gym, I looked at all kinds, both cheap and expensive. I really wanted to see that the guys behind the counter, training others, and even in maintenance CARED whether I was performing my workout safely, and to make sure I didn't need anything else to maximize my workout.

The gym I ended up deciding on (The Rush, a Southern-based chain but rapidly expanding to other areas) did just that. The PRICE of membership outweighed the COST I'd face by finding a gym that saw me as a number and risked letting me hurt myself on one of the machines or weights.

Location
Simply put, the more convenient it is to go, the better. Near your job, your home, or your kids' soccer practice - whatever! You'll come up with enough excuses on your own to get out of going if you aren't careful. Make sure location or ease of attending isn't one of them!

Hours
Here's where 24-Hour gyms shine (mine's 24 hours and I LOVE THAT!) Just knowing you can go anytime you want has a great appeal. Where do you fit in? Try your best to set a time when your minutes in the gym are honored, un-rushed and efficaciously applied. Smile. Be happy. Will you really train at 3 A.M.?

Phone contact

Don't be afraid to call ahead of time to find out just what your potential gym offers! With gas prices fluctuating, it's cheaper and easier to call in advance. I picked up the phone and found out that my gym had childcare and even a McArches-style playground! My kids now beg to go so they can play while I workout!...all from a phone call!

Membership volume (crowd)

How crowded does your prospective gym get? Visit the gym during the hours you're most likely to be working out. See how crowded both the cardio AND strength training areas are (remember, you're going to be doing both!)

Will you have to wait for machines? Do they have a variety of each machine to choose from (for example, leg curl machines, standing hamstring curl machines, and laying hamstring curl machines all work the same area - HAMSTRINGS! Having several to choose from can allow you to continue to workout even if someone is using the one you typically go to.

Amenities

Don't pay for a lap pool, giant sauna, lounge and aerobics room if you're not going to use them. More is not necessarily better and it might be necessarily more expensive. Are you easily distracted? If so, a lot of loud televisions blaring the latest doom and gloom from local news stations may not be in your cards (but they invented MP3 players and even ear plugs for a reason).

My gym even has a smoothie bar. Have I used it? Sure. If I forget my post-workout shake (don't panic, you aren't there yet. That's in the Advanced version of this book!) I'll grab a smoothie. But I prefer to know what goes into my shakes, so I usually bring one from home. That means a smoothie bar isn't a deal maker for me. But since I've used it in the past, it isn't a deal breaker either.

Equipment

I've already touched on having different machines that work the same bodypart. There also needs to be some organization, too! That means having all the arm machines in one area, leg machines in another. TRUST ME - it'll save you time from having to run from one side of the gym to the other, just to finish your workout.

I personally enjoy a wide variety of free weights (dumbbells) too. It gives me variety in my workout and allows me to move up in weight incrementally if necessary on specific body parts.

Atmosphere

This is not the mall. It's a gym. It's not a singles bar. It's a gym. It's not a childbirthing class (Guys who grunt while working out are my own personal pet peeve. HA!) It's a gym.

You won't maximize your time at the gym if you're constantly self-conscious about who you're working out next to or feeling intimidated by the guy next to you.

This is YOUR journey. You're moving at your own pace. But if you're surrounded by a bunch of gorillas flexing after each set, there are better gyms to choose from (My gym has a handful of these guys. They're funnier to watch and laugh at than anything else.)

Remember different people have different agendas at the gym. One person is there to build muscle. Another person may there to build fat. But there needs to be a nice mix.

Management Attitude

I hate to feel like I'm interrupting or bothering someone who's talking to a buddy in order to get a question answered. Some trainers can develop a "holier than thou" attitude and are put off when asked for help. At the same time, you gotta be mindful - if they're working with a client who is paying for their time, you're outta line if you step in.

However, if you aren't being treated with respect by people who are enthusiastic to help you, keep looking. (The receptionists at my gym always say, "Have a good workout" when I check in. I just love that.)

Clientele

Who's to your left, who's to your right and are they agreeable? You're coming to the gym to get lifted up, not punched down. No one wants to go to a spin class full of snobs who look down on the newbie. And a bunch of "better than yous" make getting the right weight for your next set impossible.

Chances are, people are paying you way less attention than you think they are. However, if you notice blatant rudeness in abundance, find a place you're more comfortable.

Cleanliness

Ugh. Who wants to shower after a workout in a dirty lockerroom? Who wants to lift weights after someone who literally rains sweat all over the machine?

Check out the cleanliness of the gym. Staph infections and other nasties (even the common cold) rest where germs abound. Any gym that reminds its members to clean up after themselves is a good one. Some gyms (mine included) require that people carry a towel to clean up the machines after they are used. They even sell towels at the front for those who forget! Gotta love that!

Your First Date
Make sure your club has a "trial membership". You'll wanna check it out for yourself in a "live" workout and see if it's right for you. Are there a bunch of "lookie loos" in the lockerroom? Did you enjoy a particular class more than you thought you would?

Take the time to really check out your potential gym and make sure that you're dating the future Mr. or Mrs. Gym that's right for you.

It's Not You, It's Me
You won't be able to find ALL the criteria I've laid out above in one gym without trying it out first. It's almost impossible to find a gym that doesn't want you to sign a contract. That's fine. It's common, it's expected. Just get use to that part.

However, ask what the cancellation policy of your gym is when you're talking with the sales staff. Find out what happens if you move or decide the gym isn't right for you. (Mine charges $99 to get out of my contract. A small price to pay for saving my credit score and/or having to pay for a long period of time without getting the perks of attending!)

In the end, you gotta find what works for your personality. Take the time and make this decision carefully. You're gonna be enjoying the perks of good health for a long time to come and will want to make sure the gym you choose is with you for the long haul too!

Part III - Kaizen Life

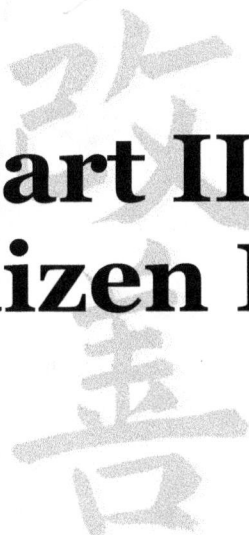

改善

Chapter 17: Realistic Goal Setting

Y ou may have tried to set goals for yourself in the past and failed. Maybe you've always been too afraid to set a goal for fear of failure.

Maybe you just haven't known what to realistically expect from your body.

Before we talk about setting your goal for weight loss success, let's look at some of the "dangers" in setting your goals too high or too low:

Setting Your Goals Too High

I'm sure you've heard by now...Nearly ninety-seven percent of all new diets started will fail.

Why is that? Do the survivors know something you don't? Have they got the inside track on what to do and how to do it? Maybe.

Who knows? The first few attempts are tough, to say the least. You try every new 'magic pill' and exercise plan under the sun. But life happens, or you get too sore from the first workout, or you realize the plan is unrealistic and leaves you feeling so hungry you're about to pass out. Most of the 'diets' out there are unrealistic and actually set you up for failure to begin with!

So what can you do? For starters, if you've gotten this far it means that you are seriously interested in increasing your chances at survival. I want to preface everything in this book with the comment that:

Unless you're willing to make small changes, you shouldn't even bother reading this.

I'm pouring my heart out and making sure that all of the things no one told me (but I wish they had) are available to you.

Secondly, I cannot guarantee your success. I can't put the right food in your mouth. I can't do the workouts for you. There are several factors outside of this book that I have no control over. You must be willing to do ALL the research necessary and even then, <u>YOU are in control</u>. No one else. Never, ever lose that thought.

Many books and seminars tell you to set goals and I couldn't agree with them more. However, if you've never set goals, (or set but never kept up with them) this is really a struggle.

So you write down what you WANT to have lost or done within a set time frame...and then miss it completely. Does this mean that you are a bad person or that you don't deserve to lose weight? Absolutely NOT!

However, it could mean that the goals you set for yourself were a little on the "lofty" side and could use some revision.

One of the reasons that unattainable goals are so detrimental to your weight loss deals with your psyche. You know, that thing that keeps you getting up in the morning, your drive, motivation, focus.

By having such goals (that are merely too high to reach in the timeframe allotted) you face the possibility of "failing". This is not to say that YOU are a failure or anything like that.

What I am saying is that you set these goals and they simply weren't reached for whatever reason. They were too high to begin with.

You might have gotten all pumped up from an infomercial or new diet pill on the market.

You might have never set goals like these before and therefore didn't know how much weight was realistic to lose in a specific amount of time.

You might have had some major setbacks in your life that kept you from reaching your full potential (stress is a mother-shutchomouth! and can sidetrack even the most motivated dieters).

Whatever the reason, you have to keep in mind that these missed goals are merely small setbacks. They aren't the end of the world and they aren't going to sneak up on you in your sleep. They can't hurt you.

Pick yourself up, reset your goals, and try again. THAT is the sign of a true businessperson.

The opposite of this mistake is just as deadly. It's setting your goals too low!

Setting Your Goals Too Low

As with the 'too high' mistake, keep in mind the words of Zig Ziglar, "Failure is an event, not a person. Yesterday ended last night. Today is a new day and it's going to be magnificent!"

Did you know that you can set yourself up for failure by setting your goals too low as well?

Nothing makes you feel better than achieving your goals. By human nature, we all want to win.

It feels good, no doubt about it. However, when the goals you set are too low or too easily attainable, things start to happen within you.

You change. You get a little cockier, a little full of yourself. You can't be touched. Then suddenly, life happens and everything comes crashing down.

It's nothing to be embarrassed about. It's happened to the best of us, I assure you. Heck, there are even some folks who speak from stage who have let success go to their heads and lose touch with reality.

So how do you combat this easily-made mistake? One thing to keep in mind is that your goals are there not only to hold you accountable, but to push you a little as well.

If you aren't being challenged by your own goals, then you are probably caught in the middle of this deadly mistake. Don't worry, no goal is set in stone. They can be fixed.

Think about it…Without challenging yourself, what fun are goals? Make sure that you have some goals that are easy to reach, no doubt about that.

Have both long and short term goals which will cause you to work a little harder, or find that motivation within yourself to get the job done. Short term goals are always fun to meet and get off the ol' "to do" list.

But when that long-term goal is met, you'll really feel a sense of pride when you can check it off your list.

Setting Realistic Goals 101

So how do you go about setting weight loss goals for yourself that don't just include "I wanna lose X pounds YESTERDAY!"

There are 3 easy steps to creating realistic goals that you can succeed with:

Step 1: Write down one specific goal, include specific dates to achieve that goal, write in present tense. Rewrite your goals often to make certain the ones that mean the most are still applicable.
Step 2: Write down all the reasons that your goal could fail.
Step 3: Write down what you can do to combat those obstacles.

Can it be that easy? Sure it is!

I've created a series of worksheets at the end of this book to help you with your goal setting. There's also a list of questions that you can print and place next to your computer, refrigerator, and anywhere else where temptation is likely to lurk. This ensures that, if an obstacle should arise, you'll be able to beat it before it even becomes an issue!

Chapter 18: How to Cut 15,640 Calories

our typical day should consist of 5-6 meals (if you're following the steps I laid out for you). But that doesn't mean that you have to live and die by the snack machine at work! Your daily caloric choices dictate whether you're gonna make it past lunch or eat your co-worker out of desperation.

Let's take a look at a typical workday for you:

Breakfast:	Kcal	Fat	Carbs	Protein
Strawberry jelly	50	0	13	0
White toast	67	.8	12.7	1.9
Egg	78	5.3	.6	6.3
Snack #1:				
Candybar	280	14	35	4

Lunch:				
Large Mac, med fries, med Coke	1130	48	151	29
Snack #2:				
Skittles candy	170	2	39	0
Dinner:				
Appetizer (Chili's chips and dip)	930	77	39	24
Salad*Cheese	111	9.5	6.8	.3
Croutons	186	7.3	25.4	4.3
Bacon bits	25	1.5	0	3
Ranch dressing	137	14.6	1.9	.3
Main Course: Fried Chicken	294	14.9	10.2	28.1
French fries	380	19	47.9	4.6
Dessert: Chocolate cake	235	10.5	34.9	2.6
Snack #3:				
Pretzels	228	1.6	47.9	6.2
Bedtime snack:				
Ice cream	780	48	79	13
Totals:	**5081**	**274**	**544**	**127.6**
x5 days a week:	**25405**	**1370**	**2720**	**638**

That's twice your recommended daily caloric intake, not to mention what you're binging on over the weekend!
*Lettuce and tomato are included in these figures

Now let's take a look at what your day COULD look like if you just swapped out a few key items and ingredients...

Breakfast:	Kcal	Fat	Carbs	Protein
Agave Nectar	15	0	4	0
Pumpernickel	19	.2	3.9	.6
Egg Whites	17	.1	.2	3.6
Snack #1:				
Apple	53	.2	13.9	.3
Lunch:				
Canned tuna, whole grain crackers, baby carrots	210	7.2	24.8	13.1
Snack #2:				
Watermelon	13	.1	3.2	.3
Dinner:				
Appetizer (bruschetta and pita from Macaroni Grill)	630	15	96	28
Salad* Avacado	47	4.4	2.4	.6
Sunflower seeds	47	4	1.9	1.5
Jalapeno	6	.2	1	.2
Balsamic vinaigrette	80	8	2	0
Main Course Grilled Chicken	180	4	0	35
Sweet potato wedges	76	0	19	1
Dessert: Cup of strawberries with chocolate syrup	146	.4	35.1	1.5
Snack #3:				
Edamame	84	3.8	6.6	7.4
Bedtime snack:				
Chocolate Casein shake with 1% milk	330	11.5	18.3	36.5

and natural peanut butter				
Totals:	**1953**	**59.1**	**232.3**	**129.6**
x5 days a week:	**9765**	**295.5**	**1161.5**	**648**
Much better! You can even have a slice of pizza or two on the weekend thanks to the attention you've paid to your meal plan during the week!				

Now, let's do the math:

	Kcal	Fat	Carbs	Protein
Poor weekly eating choices:	25405	1370	2720	638
Good weekly eating choices	9765	295.5	1161.5	648
You saved:	**15640**	**1074.5**	**1558.5**	**+10**

Wowww! And that's just ONE WEEK! Let's multiply that by 4 weeks...

	Kcal	Fat	Carbs	Protein
Poor eating choices:	101620	5480	10880	2552
Good eating choices	39060	1182	4646	2592
You saved:	**62560**	**4298**	**6234**	**+50**

That's over *four thousand grams of fat* removed from your diet in just one month! Check out the last column! You've added 50 grams of fat-burning, muscle-feeding protein to your body over the course of a month! That's fantastic!

And when you consider it takes 3,500 calories to equal one pound of fat – *you can lose up to 17 pounds* in one month, just by changing your eating habits!

A lot of "weight" is put on one's ability to get into the gym, work up a good sweat, and burn the fat. But never, ever underestimate the power of what you're eating. It could mean the difference between you working IN a cubicle…or looking like one!

To Sum It Up:
1. Choose healthier alternatives to the foods you eat to lower your "calorie bill".
2. Having small meals throughout the day minimizes your chance at binging!
3. Don't be afraid to have more protein. That's the stuff that builds your muscle and helps you burn fat faster!

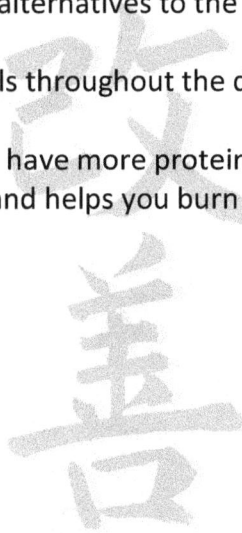

改善

Chapter 19: The Poop on Fiber

O.K boys and girls. Its time to talk about fiber!

Everyone says you need it. No one says why. Some say you need 12-24 grams of it a day (according to the British Nutrition Foundation). Others, like the United States National Academy of Sciences, Institute of Medicine say you need to ingest 20-35 grams of fiber a day.

Too much leads to bloating, cramps, and gas (just what you want when you're headed to the gym!) Too little backs you up for days.

In truth, the average American consumes less than 50% of the dietary fiber levels for good health (Source: Wikipedia).

By the time you're finished reading this article, you'll not only know why fiber is so important, but you'll also have a new appreciation for the stuff!

But in order to know how to use it to do your body good – you gotta know what it does!

Warning! Science Ahead!

For starters, fiber isn't digested by your body like fats, proteins, or carbs. In fact, it stays pretty much the same until it hits your colon.

That's where the two types of fiber come into play: those that don't dissolve in water (insoluble fiber) and those that do (soluble fiber).

First, *insoluble fiber*. This is the stuff that makes you "go". If you're dealing with constipation or do not have regular bowel movements, this is the type of fiber you're looking for! Whole-wheat flour, wheat bran, nuts and many vegetables are good sources of insoluble fiber.

While that may seem like the most important type of fiber to consume, don't forget the other, just-as-important-type of fiber, *soluble fiber*.

Think about the last time you cooked oatmeal on the stove. The 'stuff' that gives it that creamy, thick consistence we associate with oatmeal? That's soluble fiber. This type of fiber helps lower blood cholesterol and glucose levels.

Wanna help stave off pre-diabetes, heart disease, or diverticular disease? This is the stuff that does it! (I told you it was just as important as insoluble fiber!)

You can find generous quantities of soluble fiber in oats, peas, beans, apples, citrus fruits, carrots, barley and psyllium. (Source: Mayo Clinic)

C'mon and Take a Free Ride

Now that you know about the two types of fiber, let's explore what happens when you eat it! It all starts with breakfast...

Call it a moment of weakness, but let's say you have a bowl of cereal for breakfast, chocked full of refined carbohydrates.

Because these carbs are fast-digesting, they are quickly absorbed by the body – increasing the amount of sugar headed towards your liver. As your glucose levels (blood sugar) increase, it calls in an order of extra insulin from your pancreas.

Insulin is the "traffic cop" in your system that directs where the energy from the carbs should be directed.

Trouble is, after its been produced, insulin stays in your body for 5 hours! If you eat breakfast at 8am, then at lunch just 4 hours later you have a piece of cake...that sugar heads back towards your liver, creating another insulin spike. The pancreas then sends out more insulin, spiking it higher after each meal.

And what happens when you've got too much insulin in your system, kids? Insulin resistance, diabetes, and obesity (increased fat storage).

Since insulin prevents the sugar from being absorbed by your cells (cuz you have too much of it in you), it turns into fat.

Foods rich in fiber practice the 'buddy system' and will break down more slowly in your system, not giving you the insulin spike we spoke of earlier. Because they're absorbed gradually, your body can better process them (and you feel fuller longer to boot!)

For example, a large salad, even when coupled with a cream-based dressing like Ranch or Thousand Island, will not increase your blood sugar.

However, many grains, like rice, barley, rye, and corn can increase your blood sugar, even though they are 'complex carbohydrates' (those 'buddy system' carbs noted earlier).

This can happen if a large serving is eaten quickly without having oils or proteins in your meal. You knew there was a reason your mother always told you to chew your food slowly!

The Lighter Side of Fiber

So far, we've seen the damage your body can undergo via a lack of fiber. And as if battling obesity wasn't a big enough reason (pun intended) – here are some more benefits to consuming the right amount of fiber!

Benefit #1 – Lower Risk of Heart Disease: Mentioned earlier in this article, fiber lowers cholesterol. It's been well documented that a buildup of cholesterol in the coronary arteries leads to atherosclerosis (hardening of the arteries). They become hard and narrow. Should they become blocked altogether, this produces a heart attack.

In fact, in a Harvard study of over 40,000 male health professionals, researchers found that a high total dietary fiber intake was linked to a 40 percent lower risk of coronary heart disease, compared to a low fiber intake.

Benefit #2 – Decreased risk for Type 2 Diabetes: Remember our trip down Insulin Lane earlier? Type 2 diabetes is the most common form of diabetes. When the body develops the insulin resistance we previously discussed, type 2 diabetes is the result.

When it comes to factors that increase the risk of developing diabetes, a diet low in cereal fiber and rich in high-glycemic-index foods (which cause big spikes in blood sugar) seems particularly bad.

One Harvard study of more than 700,000 men and women, found that eating an extra 2 servings of whole grains a day decreased the risk of type 2 diabetes by 21 percent. (Source: Harvard School of Public Health)

Benefit #3 – Lower Risk of Diverticular Disease: Betcha didn't even know you were at risk on this one!

Typically an inflammation of the intestine, studys show that this diease occurs in one-third of all those over age 45 and in two-thirds of those over age 85. (Source: Harvard School of Public Health)

Among male health professionals in a long-term follow-up study, eating dietary fiber, particularly insoluble fiber, was associated with about a 40 percent lower risk of diverticular disease.

Benefit #4 – Go More Often: **Duh!** Probably the most well-known benefit of fiber is that it relieves constipation! The good news is that your GI (gastrointestinal) tract is highly sensitive to dietary fiber and if you're backed up, fiber will put the steam back in your locomotive!

If you're truly having difficulty? Go for wheat or oat bran. It's been found to be more effective than fruits and veggies.

But don't go 'whole hog' on fiber! There are distinct disadvantages to taking in too much, too soon!

Too Much of a Good Thing?
Just as with sweets and chocolates, you gotta think 'moderation' here. There are actual consequences for bulking up on fiber too quickly!

1. **Constipation** - eating the right amount of foods rich in fiber can help with any 'traffic jams' in the bathroom. However, fiber absorbs water. Eating too much fiber without drinking plenty of water can have the opposite of its intended effect! Don't forget your eight to ten 8oz glasses of water a day in addition to slowly increasing your fiber intake!

2. **Gas** - increased flatulence is a very common side effect of high-fiber diet. Once the fiber hits your colon, bacteria begin to chow down, doing what they can to digest it – creating bloating and gas as a byproduct. Sadly, this occurs regardless of the type of fiber you're eating, so be sure to grab a little Beano before you chow down on your next bowl of oatmeal!

3. **Deprivation of good cholesterol** - while it is true that high fiber diet is effective in lowering cholesterol, not all

cholesterol is bad. In fact, according to research, high-density lipoprotein (HDL) is effective in protecting the heart and brain. Eating more than the recommended daily amount of fiber may reduce both types of cholesterol from the blood.

Foods rich in fiber are not bad, rather healthful. However, too much of anything good can be bad.

Yum – Paper Sandwich!

Fiber doesn't have to taste like cardboard! There are some really yummy options to getting the proper amount of fiber your body needs to perform like the well-oiled machine you know it can be!

1. **Go with whole fruit instead of juice.** Whole apples and whole oranges are packed with a lot more fiber and a lot fewer calories than their liquid counterparts.
2. **Break the fast with fruit.** Get off to a great start by adding fruit, like berries or melon, to your breakfast every day.
3. **Check the label for fiber-filled whole grains.** Choose foods that list whole grains (like whole wheat or whole oats) as a first ingredient. Bread, cereal, crackers and other grain foods should have at least 3 grams of fiber per serving. Read "Health Gains from Whole Grains" for a list of whole grains and their benefits.
4. **Eat more beans.** It's easy to forget about beans, but they're a great tasting, cheap source of fiber, good carbs, protein, and other important nutrients.
5. **Try a new dish.** Test out international recipes that use whole grains, like tabouli or whole wheat wheat pasta, or beans, like Indian dahls.

Armed with the proper knowledge (and a better understanding of WHY and HOW fiber works so well) you can now make more informed decisions on giving your body the nutrients, minerals, and supplements it needs to run at your pace!

Chapter 20: Worksheets

F ind something interesting that you don't wanna re-create yourself? As with the rest of this book, my goal is to see you succeed, so I want you to use what I've already created to lose the weight and let nothing stand in your way. On the following pages are worksheets mentioned throughout the book that you can reprint and use over and over again.

And please, let me know if there's anything else you'd like to know about, feel like I've left out, or would like to see in future updates of this book by emailing me at Rachel@whatifyouwerethin.com.

Have you used this book to lose weight? Is there something you're struggling with and want my help to overcome? Got some before and after pix of your own you'd like to share? Lemme know!

I'm always listening and look forward to hearing of your successes!

Daily Food Diary

Food	Calories	Protein	Carbs	Fat
Breakfast				
TOTAL				
Mid-morning snack				
TOTAL				
Lunch				
TOTAL				
Mid-afternoon/Post-workout Snack				
TOTAL				
Dinner				
TOTAL				
Daily Total				
Daily Allowance				
Results				

Did you drink 8-10 8oz glasses of water today?	How much?

Commercial Break Program Checklist (check each exercise off as you complete it)

Exercise	30 sec	1 min	1:30	2 min	2:30	3 min
March in place						
Shoulder touches						
Toe touches						
Adductor squeeze						
Warrior 1						
Side lunge						

改善

Four Minute Fitness (check each exercise off as you complete it)

Exercise	Mon	Tues	Wed	Thurs	Fri
March in place					
Jumping jacks					
Squat and press					
Forward lunge and hammer curl					
Anterior raise with side lunge					
Plank					

Easy Office Fitness (check each exercise off as you complete it)

Exercise	Mon	Tues	Wed	Thurs	Fri
New Idea					
Nothing, why?					
Goofing off					
Just stretching my legs					
No fake reason needed					
Another invisible move					

改善

Goal Setting Worksheet

Goal:	Obstacle Preventing Goal:	Overcome it by:

改善

Daily Questions to Keep You on Track:

1. Will eating what I have in my hand get me closer to my goals? (If yes, eat it. If not, "weigh" the consequences!)
2. Am I doing everything I can most days to work on my health? If not, where can I improve?
3. If today was a workout day, did I do something to increase my fitness level?
4. How am I feeling about my progress? What can I do to pass on this good feeling to others?
5. When I look in the mirror, what's one thing I can say that I LOVE about myself?

Binge Buster: Write the pros and cons of what you want to splurge on to see if its really worth it!

Food in Question:	I want to eat it because:	Is this a pro or con to my weight loss goal?

Email me at <u>rachel@racheldyoung.com</u> and I will send you a printable version of the following two pages and place them in either places you'll face temptation (in order to keep your urges at bay) or to remind you of your goals.

I place my "Stop Sign" on the refrigerator, kitchen cabinets, and keep a small one in my wallet next to my credit card for times when I want to buy something sweet that I shouldn't.

I keep my "Answer" sign next to my workout equipment, my gym shoes, and workout DVDs.

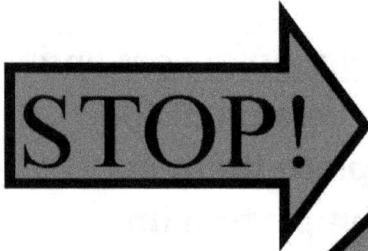
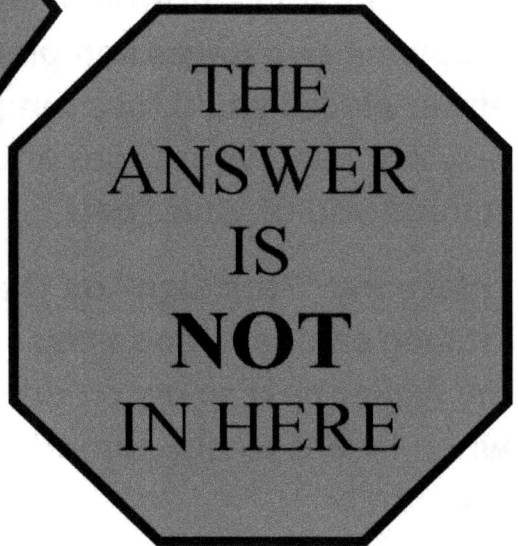

THE
ANSWER
IS
NOT
IN HERE

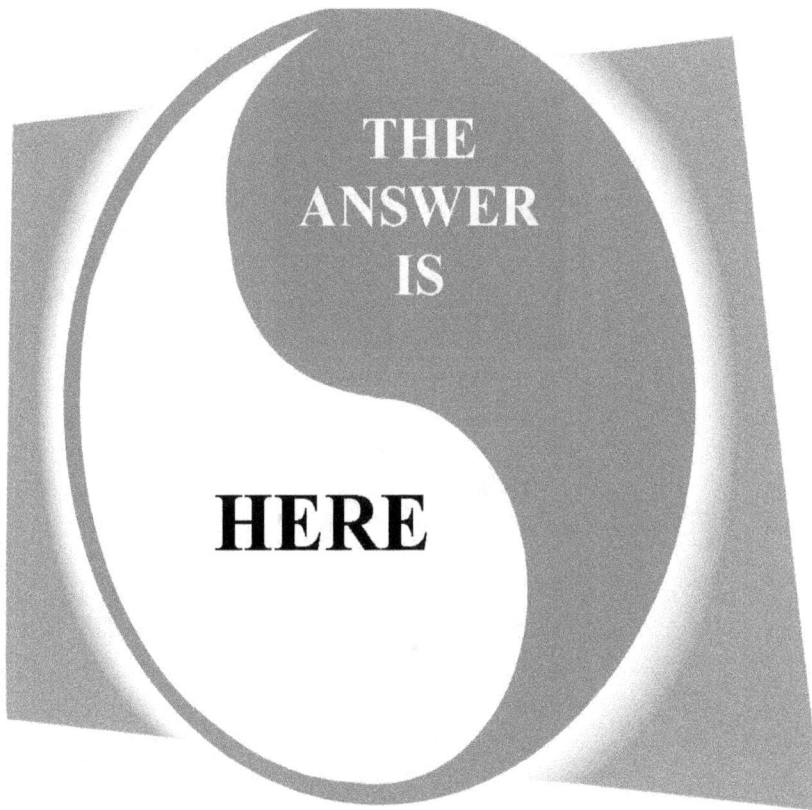

改善

Chapter 21: To Sum It Up (Combined)

ere's a summary of the material you've just read. Feel free to print it out and post it somewhere that you can go back to it when you need to!

Chapter 2:

1. You didn't get this way overnight and won't lose the weight overnight. Be patient!

2. This is about changing your lifestyle, one step at a time. Don't do anything radical or it won't "stick"!

3. Don't worry. I'm gonna be here the whole way to help you out. Remember, I went through this 80 pounds ago and know exactly what you're going through!

Chapter 5:

1. If you can't reduce the stress in your life (or find a better way to handle it), you'll have a hard time losing the last few pounds due to cortisol.
2. Artificial sweeteners create an illusion within the body that insulin is needed and can eventually cause "insulin resistance" (and lead to diabetes).
3. There's no such thing as "zero calories" – regardless of what the label says!

Chapter 6:

1. Look for "clean" food – if you can't pronounce its ingredients, can't grow it, pick it, or get it cut lean from your butcher, don't eat it!
2. You're human. Birthday cake is ok as long as it's only a slice and only a rare occasion.
3. Cut your grocery bill by buying fresh and eating in rather than paying someone else to cook for you!

Chapter 8:

1. "When" to eat is just as important as "what" to eat!
2. If you're in the Beginner Stage, eat breakfast to begin your kaizen transformation. It jumpstarts your metabolism and increases your energy for the day!
3. Chew your food slowly and enjoy what you're eating. Food is no longer the enemy!
4. Eat 5-6 meals a day to rev up your metabolism and keep from binging when you get hungry.
5. Drink more water. You'll feel fuller, have an easier time in the bathroom, and your skin will even look better!
6. As you advance, eat your starchy carbs towards the

beginning of the day to keep your insulin levels down and your energy up, up, up!

Chapter 9:

1. Indulge yourself – But throw out the first bite!
2. No substitutions for your sugary favs with its sugar-free alternative. Don't let your mind think its ok to still eat garbage!
3. If you can't control yourself, then don't bring it home. If you know you'll eat it all in one sitting, then don't buy it at all.
4. Drink water, buy smaller plates, eat smaller meals more often, and stay away from gum to reduce cravings!
5. Cheating is ok on your "cheat meal day". One meal, once a week. No more. No less!

Chapter 10:

1. Matchbox-sized cheese portions keep the fat content to a minimum.
2. Eat as much of the carbs as you want (but keep your fruit intake to a minimum – no more than 5oz at a meal)!
3. Read the recommended portion size on the side of the nutrition label to ensure you're eating the right amount!

Chapter 11:

1. Once you're advanced enough to track your caloric intake, get a notebook and write down everything you put in your mouth to see just how much you've "really" been eating!
2. Eat before you go grocery shopping to avoid unnecessary purchases.
3. Keep your salads interesting by varying the types of ingredients you choose!

Chapter 18:

1. Choose healthier alternatives to the foods you eat to lower your "calorie bill".
2. Having small meals throughout the day minimizes your chance at binging!
3. Don't be afraid to have more protein. That's the stuff that builds your muscle and helps you burn fat faster!

Take Your Weight Loss Journey to a Whole New Level!

If you'd like to jump start your weight loss success, visit us online at:

www.WhatIfYouWereThin.com

where you can receive instant access to:

- ✓ Weekly meal plans and matching grocery lists created by a Registered Dietician, specific for the amount of weight YOU want to lose!
- ✓ Weekly strength-training workouts designed by a professional female fitness model to keep your workouts fresh and invigorating!
- ✓ Weekly Latin and Hip-Hop workout videos to sculpt your body in fun, exciting ways!
- ✓ Don't forget about the monthly newsletter delivered straight to your email inbox with tips, tricks, and new techniques to make weight loss fun and exciting!

What are you waiting for?

改善

www.ingramcontent.com/pod-product-compliance
Lightning Source LLC
Chambersburg PA
CBHW050127280326
41933CB00010B/1275